BAGUA DAOYIN

BAGUA DAOYIN

A UNIQUE BRANCH OF DAOIST LEARNING:
A Secret Skill of the Palace

HE JINGHAN

TRANSLATED BY DAVID ALEXANDER

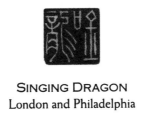

SINGING DRAGON
London and Philadelphia

First published in English in 2008
by Singing Dragon
An imprint of Jessica Kingsley Publishers
116 Pentonville Road
London N1 9JB, UK
and
400 Market Street, Suite 400
Philadelphia, PA 19106, USA

www.singing-dragon.com

First published in Chinese by Lion Books in 2002
Copyright © He Jinghan 2008
English translation copyright © David Alexander 2008
Original Chinese edition copyright © Lion Books 2002

Library of Congress Cataloging in Publication Data
He, Jinghan.
  Bagua Daoyin : a unique branch of Daoist learning, a secret skill of the palace / He Jinghan ; translated by David Alexander ; foreword by Paul Alexander.
    p. cm.
  ISBN 978-1-84819-009-2 (pb : alk. paper)
  1. Martial arts--Psychological aspects. 2. Tai chi. 3. Exercise. 4. Mind and body. I. Alexander, David. II. Title.
  GV1102.7.P75J56 2008
  796.815--dc22
                              2008014955

British Library Cataloguing in Publication Data
A CIP catalogue record for this book is available from the British Library

ISBN 978 1 84819 009 2

Printed and bound in Great Britain by
Athenaeum Press, Gateshead, Tyne and Wear

CONTENTS

FOREWORD – AN INTRODUCTION TO HE JINGHAN AND BAGUA QUAN

I first met Master He Jinghan in the summer of 2003 and it was then that I decided to learn Bagua Quan.

Every movement of every exercise has a specific purpose. The system is designed to go from simple to complex, carrying the practitioner into the depths of the Bagua Quan system.

With every physical concept that is presented within the forms and movements of the Bagua Quan system, there is also a philosophical one.

Within the Bagua Quan system are many sub-systems – some for health, others for combat.

I have studied for only a short time – but I have researched the exercises in practice and I have tried to integrate the philosophical and physical concepts into my life. My body, mind and life have changed a great deal for the better.

Bagua Quan exercises develop the self and guide you to build a foundation and discover every part of your body. Starting with opening the skeletal frame, the muscles and joints, the exercises lead inward to the tendons, ligaments, fascia, organs and the mind.

Bagua Quan is indeed a rare Chinese martial art. But the benefits of Bagua Quan practice are not just combative skill – the real treasure is the depth and clarity of the principles, principles that can lead you to better your posture, regulate the blood flow and release the restrictions that tension can cause in the body.

Bagua Quan is an ancient martial art practice, originating in the timeless mountains of China. Developed from Chinese philosophy, Daoist health practices and classical Chinese martial arts, it became well known in the mid 1800s via Master Dong Haichuan who taught at the Imperial Palace. His disciple Yin Fu carried the art to the next generation within the Forbidden City in the early 1900s. Masters Gong Baoshan and Gong Baotian brought the art from the palace to their home town – Qingshan Village.

Master Gong Baozhai also came from Qingshan village and so was raised in a community of Bagua Quan practitioners. He settled in Taiwan in the 1940s and started to transmit Bagua Quan to a small group of disciples.

He Jinghan spent 25 years living with Master Gong Baozhai and in this book he shares some of his passion and understanding of the ancient art of Bagua Quan.

It is a system not only of great combative resource but perhaps more importantly in these modern times, it is a system of health exercises that can open and connect the body, that can help the practitioner to keep a balanced mind and live in this fast-changing world by looking inside ourselves – body and mind – to discover how and why we move and think the way we do.

I believe that this book is of great importance to us all. Master He Jinghan has successfully brought concepts of an ancient world into our modern times and now with the help of my father, David Alexander, and Singing Dragon books – to a Western audience.

Paul Alexander
24th March 2008

TRANSLATOR'S INTRODUCTION

I first became involved with He Jinghan's work two year's ago when my son, Paul, asked me to translate the captions of the photographs in this book to help with his own Bagua Quan training. After doing this I browsed through the book out of curiosity and became encaptivated by He Jinghan's cultured prose and his stories of his own early life and about his master Gong Baozhai. Reading on into his explanation of Bagua Daoyin I realised that this was a significant work. Its translation become a labour of love for me and with its publication I feel privileged to have played a part in bringing He Jinghan's teachings to a wider audience.

Although a Chinese translator for many years I previously had little experience of Chinese martial arts. I have greatly benefited from He Jinghan's advice, especially in the chapters on the inner theory of Bagua Quan. However any inaccuracies or infelicities in this translation are solely my responsibility.

I have tried to capture the style of He Jinghan's writing. This is cultured, erudite, and analytic but with touches of down to earth humour. This can be challenging at times, especially when he displays his deep knowledge of Chinese culture with quotations from the classics, but it is always a pleasure to read.

The translator of Chinese martial arts texts often faces a quandary with specialised terminology. Should this be translated idiomatically into Englishor literally, so keeping some of the original flavour of the Chinese, or should the term be left in transliterated Chinese which at least does not distort the meaning? The 'quan' of Bagua Quan is a case in point. It literally means 'fist' or 'boxing' but its wider meaning is 'a system of martial arts'. So should Bagua Quan be translated as 'eight trigrams boxing' or 'the branch of martial arts based on the Bagua system', or left as it is as a widely recognised term? And what about Sixiang Quan and Bazhang Quan? There is no 'correct' answer.

I have followed the line of keeping a term in its transliterated (Pinyin) form when it is well known (e.g. Daoyin, Taiji, Qi, Yin, Yang) but otherwise translating into the nearest English term, even though this may be imprecise – e.g. shape (xing), potential force (shi), spirit (shen), intent (yi), force (li)).

For the terms retained in their original form I have included a glossary giving the basic meaning.

GLOSSARY

Bagua	Eight trigram signs
Bagua Quan	Bagua martial arts style
Baguazhang	Bagua palms
Bamuzhang	Eight mother palms
Bazhang	Eight palms
Bazhang Quan	Bazhang martial arts style
Daoyin	Direct and guide
Liangyi	Two rituals
Sixiang	Four images
Qi	Basic energy
Yin Yang	Two primal opposing but complementary principles said to be found in all objects and processes in the universe

The Treasure
that Belongs to You

Bagua Daoyin is part of the training methods of Bagua Quan internal skill (neigong). It originated from the refinement of Daoist studies into training the body and mind. It was subsequently adopted by the Qing imperial court but did not spread to the outside world until the final years of the Qing dynasty when my master's master, Gong Baotian, a fourth degree swordsman bodyguard in the Qing court, retired and returned to his village. Through my master, Gong Baozhai, it was transmitted to me to meet the challenge of a new era.

My master was born six years before the republic (1905). Although he grew up in the republic he had from boyhood received an education in the scholar way and the martial way from teachers of the imperial era – he was a man who straddled both eras, half old and half new. However, his way of imparting knowledge of Bagua Quan was traditional. He would say 'it is extremely tiring for a martial arts master to have pupils everywhere under the sun. It would be an insult to the master. It is no compliment, it just shows that not a single one would be well taught. It would be amazing if a master could teach as many as five disciples in his lifetime; he would die from exhaustion. How could so many be taught?' It could certainly not be done following the methods that my master used to teach me.

I was born in 1955, half a century after my master. This is a completely different age. The forces of production in all branches of industry are enormous. There is a continuous stream of new products. Only a handful of eccentrics keep to the old 'traditional' ways. If these old ways have no commercial value then only people like myself who are fated to do so will get involved in them. Yet they should not be thrown away. I have been involved in martial arts for over thirty years, starting out of curiosity then gradually becoming fascinated by its gracefulness and profundity. Progressing from it being a leisure activity to it becoming the main part of my life, from it being a health exercise to discovering that it is an enormous treasure, the process of transformation is really difficult to describe. I am like an explorer excavating an ancient ruin and discovering a fortress very deep underground. When I finally complete the excavation and leave the fortress to make the joyful announcement to the world I discover that many people do not understand what I am saying.

Chinese martial arts have been isolated from the present age for too long; the misunderstandings are too deep. It is like a soldier who has been discharged from the army after fighting at close quarters on the battlefield to protect his home and country. Unfortunately, he has been defeated and people now cold shoulder him and discriminate against him, leaving him to perish. The soldier shouts 'Before I went to war I was a scholar, have you forgotten? I can still help you. I am one of you.' However, the people are absorbed by the victor's aura, they watch his every movement, they pay attention to the victor's attitude. Nobody hears the soldier's cry.

Many old masters say 'If the heritage of past generations is not handed down, so be it. I can do nothing.' 'Can't the attitude be changed so that most people will want to see?' The old masters watch over the fortress and know it like the palms of their hands. They feel deeply about it and would rather that the fortress were buried again than to see a single blade of grass or a tree in it suffer damage.

The popularization of Taiji Quan is an example of what makes them grieve. 'Taiji Quan has been spoilt'. It is as if they had seen somebody use a Song dynasty palace porcelain bowl to hold dog and cat food. Taiji Quan is a very high level martial art. Soft and hard, slow, it also carries steel in its softness, uninterruptedly. The large and small tendons are exercised together in synchrony. If the body does not move extremely agilely and smoothly, operating freely, it will not succeed. But now that it has become a popular exercise everyone can do a bit of Taiji Quan and many of its fine and delicate aspects have been lost. If the worst comes to the worst it will be carried away in its coffin. Although this may be inevitable it is nevertheless a matter of regret.

But what is to be done in this age of ours? My master spent over twenty years passing on the heritage to me, a person half living in the old times. I enjoyed the training and absorbed it unconsciously. In this age how many people could devote twenty years of their lives to each other in this way? If Bagua Quan is really of no use to the people of today's world then let it die away. But in reality it is not like that. Bagua Quan not only has use, it is perhaps the most effective way to redemption for the people of today. It is just that most people do not recognise it. So this is my duty – to enable everyone to recognise it. Bagua Daoyin is the first step.

This is an age of pictures. People are used to using pictures when they speak and when they read. Martial arts were originally pictorial. The oldest and most direct method of teaching was pictorial. Very well, we will return to the essence of pictorial martial arts. This book is the first step.

Looking and admiring is to enjoy, observing is to study. I hope that this book which uses pictures as its main method of teaching can satisfy both of these objectives. If there is understanding then this treasure house will be yours. It can create a new world for you, for me and for everyone and create a new enlightened majority for the world so that martial arts will be able to move forward to a new future.

He Jinghan

CHAPTER 1

Bagua,
Bagua Quan and
Bagua Daoyin

BAGUA

The Bagua are eight symbols called trigrams (gua) which are said to date back to the era of Fu Xi 4,500 years ago.

These eight symbols are

☰ ☷ ☳ ☵ ☶ ☴ ☲ ☱

Each symbol is composed of three lines which are developed and read from bottom to top. There are two types of lines, one ▬▬ which was later called the Yang line; the other ▬ ▬ which was later called the Yin line.

It is said that Fu Xi surveyed heaven and earth, the mountains and the rivers, the birds and the beasts, men and women. He deduced the characteristics of all of nature's works and used the Bagua symbols as representations. In Fu Xi's era there was no written language. Men of learning in later times produced written explanations of the symbols and gave them names.

☰ Qian   ☳ Zhen

☷ Kun   ☴ Xun

☵ Kan   ☶ Gen

☲ Li   ☱ Dui

Later each symbol came to represent different objects according their Yin and Yang characteristics and their form of generation. For example:

Name	Nature	Direction	Family	Animal	Body
Qian	Heaven	Northwest	Father	Lion	Head
Kun	Earth	Southwest	Mother	Chilin	Stomach
Kan	Water	North	Middle son	Snake	Kidney
Li	Fire	South	Middle daughter	Phoenix	Heart
Zhen	Thunder	East	Eldest son	Dragon	Liver
Xun	Wind	Southeast	Eldest daughter	Roc	Waist/lower back
Gen	Mountain	Northeast	Youngest son	Tiger	Back
Dui	Lake	South	Youngest daughter	Monkey	Lungs

Men of learning also produced two fundamental methods of arrangement of the Bagua based on the differences in their corresponding relationship. One is called 'Pre-Heaven Bagua' or 'Fu Xi Bagua' and is used to show the laws of nature. The other is called 'Post-Heaven Bagua' or 'King Wen Bagua' and is used to show applied changes in things. Subsequently the eight trigrams (gua), which were originally separate and independent, became a single entity called the Bagua. After this the concepts of the Sixiang, the Liangyi, Taiji and Wuji gradually developed.

As to the Iching (Book of Changes), this uses six symbols, produced by reduplicating two trigrams, to explain more complex changes in things.

BAGUA QUAN

Bagua Quan is a development of Chinese martial arts. Its origin is unclear but I think that it must be a Daoist system.

Bagua Quan and the Bagua are related to the twin aspects of 'internal cultivation' and 'external application'.

In the matter of internal cultivation Bagua Quan uses the principles of the Bagua to distinguish between and exercise eight parts of the body:

> heart, liver, lungs and kidneys
> (the corresponding internal trigrams are Li, Zhen, Dui and Kan)

> head, back, waist/lower back and stomach
> (the corresponding external trigrams are Qian, Gen, Xun and Kun)

In the matter of external application Bagua Quan, using the attributes of Yin and Yang, groups martial arts moves and postures into eight categories:

> Yin Yin Yin, Yin Yin Yang, Yin Yang Yang, Yin Yang Yin,

> Yang Yang Yang, Yang Yang Yin, Yang Yin Yin, Yang Yin Yang

(Basically Yin is force exerted downwards and Yang is force exerted upwards).

However all the internally cultivated parts of the body and externally applied categories of movement are interrelated in accordance with Yin and Yang changes of the Bagua.

In other words every move in Bagua Quan must conform with the principles of the Bagua and at the same time have two functions – internally to nourish life and externally to resist the opponent.

For this reason the Bagua Quan school of martial arts is named after the Bagua.

DAOYIN

The meaning of 'Daoyin' is 'to open up a pathway to allow movement to flow'; for example to open up a channel to direct the flow of water or open up a road to direct the flow of traffic. 'Daoyin' therefore implies three things:

- to open up a pathway
- to direct and guide energy
- the true direction

The art of Daoyin originated long ago in China and was already well developed and widespread in the Spring and Autumn and Warring States periods. It was a sort of stretching movement and a coordination of thought and breathing to free up the muscles and bones and open up the flow of the Qi and blood. In later years it was written about by practitioners of Daoism and comprehensively developed.

BAGUA DAOYIN

There are two stages in the 'internal cultivation and external practice' of the Bagua Quan system. The first is 'guiding Qi by force', the second is 'driving force by Qi'.

The method used in the first stage is Daoyin. 'Force' (li) comes from specific limb movements. Through the stretching and the opening and closing of the body, the skeletal and muscular connections create different 'pathways' to 'direct and guide' the energy of the Qi into eight parts of the body — the heart, liver, lungs, kidneys, head, back, waist/lower back and stomach.

Unlike the ordinary art of Daoyin, Bagua Daoyin as part of Bagua Quan is a branch of martial arts. Bagua Daoyin is not only effective in building up and nurturing the body but also trains the power and postures needed for self defence, achieving the objective of 'the combination of internal and external cultivation'. So Bagua Daoyin in addition to helping martial arts practitioners also has many other benefits. This is why I especially advocate and promote Bagua Daoyin.

CHAPTER 2

Bagua Daoyin, the Guiding Principle of Bagua

You have stretched yourself out. Your body has held a position for too long and your limbs want to spread out. Do you remember this feeling? All your muscles are tingling and your internal organs are nice and warm. This is Daoyin.

The practice of Daoyin originated in China long ago. Manuscripts unearthed from Han dynasty tombs have Daoyin illustrations. The Daoist philosopher Zhuangzi in his work 'Great Master' said 'a true person's breath goes down to his heel', which is an early reference to Daoyin. This is an important clue since stretching exercises and soft hard exercises are not solely Chinese. The Chinese are not the only people who exercise by stretching. But why was it only the Chinese who developed the practice of Daoyin?

The Chinese believe that the two basic elements that maintain the body are Qi and blood. If we can maintain the free circulation of Qi and blood, the body will be naturally healthy. The purpose of the art of Daoyin is to direct the circulation of Qi and blood by means of movements which stretch and guide the body. So there is a great difference between Daoyin and soft hard training that just exercises muscles and tendons.

Qi and blood flow in a set direction; this direction is determined by the movements stretching and guiding the body. For example when an official goes on an inspection tour he has a guide to lead him. A car is guided in a particular direction, a hydraulic engineer when dredging a river must first know in which direction the water is going. Each movement in the art of Daoyin has a definite direction. The body following this direction links up into the unified smooth internal force. The Qi and the blood therefore follow this energy and flow towards the direction determined by the use of Daoyin.

Bagua Quan's internal cultivation trains a person according to eight divisions. These eight divisions correspond to eight trigrams. In this system of inner cultivation the organs

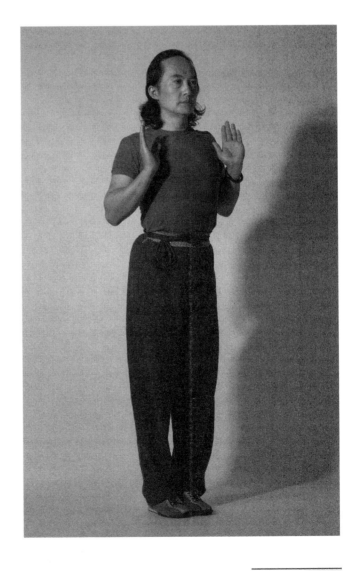

This is the 'starting posture' to control breathing. Before beginning an exercise we use 'breath control' to regulate the inner organs, Qi and blood to their normal state.

are the source of Daoyin, the arteries are the pathways of Daoyin and movements guide the direction of Daoyin. This is the deeply layered art of Daoyin.

The art of Daoyin combines keeping fit, martial arts and medical science. Its effectiveness has been proven through countless generations. In order to emphasise that it directs and guides (daoyin) the functioning of the body and to reduce the barrier between this ancient functional method and people of the present day, I have called it Bagua Daoyin. Using Daoyin everyone can be guided into the temple of health, happiness and ancient knowledge.

CHAPTER 3

Interview with
Master He Jinghan

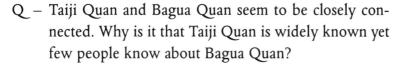

Bagua Daoyin is a body development system of boundless refinement. Those who have not yet experienced Bagua Daoyin may feel that it is impossible to enter through its gates. We have compiled this interview to encapsulate the questions that an ordinary person might ask – to cast a stone to find the way, to glimpse into the innermost recesses of Bagua Daoyin.

Q – Taiji Quan and Bagua Quan seem to be closely connected. Why is it that Taiji Quan is widely known yet few people know about Bagua Quan?

A – Bagua Quan originated in Daoism. It was not until the middle years of the Qing dynasty, when Dong Haichuan gained a reputation as a master, that Bagua Quan emerged into the open world. However the subsequent three generations of masters – Dong Haichuan, Yin Fu and Gong Baotian – all worked within the confines of the Qing palace and it was not until the final years of the Qing dynasty when Gong Baotian retired and returned to his village that Bagua Quan emerged from the imperial palace the open world.

Q – So Bagua Quan was a secret passed on within the imperial palace? Could that be why it has been more difficult to popularise than Taiji Quan?

A – Each branch of martial arts has its own difficult aspects. Bagua Quan is very fine and is also very powerful in its application. In particular the system transmitted by my master is both comprehensive and huge.

Q – As I understand it you are the fifth transmitter, and it was only with you that Bagua Quan's 'bag of secrets' was made public. So how can the ordinary person who has no foundation in martial arts study Bagua Quan?

A – The real 'bag of secrets' will not be understood by the ordinary person. However, no matter whether you are a high grade martial artist or an ordinary person, you will still use the same body framework. So the basic methods of operating the body are similar. Some basic movements practice these methods. These are very important initial steps which everyone can practice and everyone should practice. This is also the basis of the Bagua Daoyin which I present.

Q – What is the emphasis of Bagua Daoyin? Is it like the Qi of Taiji Quan?

A – Bagua Quan is the result of developing Chinese martial arts to a very high level so that what makes it up is a combination of Daoyin and Qigong and martial arts skills and it concentrates on simultaneously cultivating the internal and the external. The system of Bagua Quan is fine as well as huge. Bagua Daoyin is part of Bagua Quan's internal cultivation.

Q – Are you saying that learning Bagua Quan includes combining all these things?

A – Some of the older generation in fact felt this way. However after practicing Bagua Quan they came to feel that other martial arts did not satisfy them. So in the past very few practitioners of Bagua Quan simultaneously trained in other martial arts while many practitioners of other martial arts simultaneously trained in Bagua Quan.

Q – At what age did you start to practice martial arts?

A – I started practicing Yang style Taiji Quan when I was fifteen. When I was twenty-three I met my master and began to specialize in Bagua.

Q – From your twenty to thirty years of experience how would you advise an ordinary person to start? Is there an initial stage? For example Taiji Quan has a 24-step form, 37-step form, 42-step form right up to 108.

A – There are many schools of Taiji Quan, some new, some old. But that is not the important point. In the past martial arts were a life or death skill, not a competitive recreation, so that practicing a martial art was a matter of surviving in combat through the effective use of your body. But if you are to use your body effectively you must first become aware of your body.

Q – Become aware of your body. So can practicing Bagua Daoyin enable you to become aware of your body? You just now referred to Bagua Quan as being very fine. In what way is it fine?

A – When we learn to develop limb movements we progress from big muscles to small muscles, from large joints to small joints. When we develop martial arts skills it is also like this. From large muscle and joint exercises to small muscle and joint exercises.

Q – Could you explain what are large muscles and joints?

A – For example, when we first start to learn how to exercise our limbs as a child we use our shoulder joints and our calf muscles. These are large joints and muscles.

They are strong and easy to use. But when a child learns to eat with chopsticks and to write with a pen the fine muscles of the fingers are involved. These muscles are more flexible but need greater skill to use and develop later. This in fact is also the sequence for martial arts training which applies to everyone.

Q – So, although Bagua Quan appears to be very specialized, everyone can benefit from its body development aspects.

A – No matter whether you want to develop your body, practice martial arts or any other exercise, the important question is whether your method of exercise is correct, whether it is the most effective. So is Bagua Daoyin just a way in which people can practice how to effectively use their body? When you have learnt it you can use your body to take on any activity; it helps with everything.

Q – You just now referred to shoulders. Could you explain how to effectively use your shoulders?

A – Most people think that the arms start from the shoulders. In fact the shoulders have two locations. Close up to the neck there is the area which takes the load when we are carrying something heavy – or stretch to take out our wallet. However the arm in fact starts at the shoulder blade in the back; this enables the arm to stretch across the body. So if we want to use the arm effectively we must first effectively use the shoulder blade. But this part of the body has for a long time been overlooked by most people.

Q – So the arm can be thought of as similar to a chicken's wing.

A – This is a very good analogy. The root of a chicken's wing is like a human shoulder blade. When a chicken flaps its wings it uses this part.

Q – Normally we only occasionally use the shoulder blade. However, can basic training in Bagua Daoyin open out the numerous parts of the body which we have neglected?

A – We consider that the body has four main joints, the two shoulder blades and the two hip joints. These are the key joints that connect the four limbs to the body. When you begin Bagua Daoyin you will certainly open up these joints.

Q – How does opening up these four joints benefit us?

A – Joints enable us to move easily. However, they can degenerate if they are immobilized for a long time or if their turning range is restricted. This can affect not only movement but also the circulation of the Qi and the blood. So when we open up a joint and enlarge the gap in a joint and its range of movement it makes it easier for us to move smoothly.

Q – The Taiji Quan that we usually see seems flexible and agile, as if the body had no bones, but has a limited range of joint movements. Would it be improved if it were combined with the joint movements of Bagua Daoyin?

A – Although I have long specialized in Bagua, I have practiced and studied Taiji Quan for over thirty years. In particular practicing Bagua Quan has deepened my anatomical understanding of Taiji Quan to a degree that would not ordinarily have been possible. To sum up, even if you do not practice martial arts, if you open up your joints, you will, at the very least, give yourself a lively and free body.

Q – So is the purpose of practicing martial arts to give your body the means for greater freedom and self control?

A — My master said that the purpose in practicing martial arts was to seek a state of freedom and ease, so that we should develop towards a state of freedom and ease within our body and mind and in our relations with others.

Q — The state of freedom and ease that you speak of seems closely linked to the adaptability and resilience of the body and mind. This seems completely incompatible with the attitude which is prevalent nowadays of 'I can do anything that I want to do'. Could you elaborate on this?

A — Confucius said 'when following the directions of the mind, do not transgress what is right'. This 'following the direction of the mind' is a state of freedom and ease. But it takes place within the framework of a set of rules. As far as our body is concerned, the degree of turn of the neck determines the field of vision. If you have difficulty in turning your neck, your field of vision will not be free and you will not be able to see what you want to see. Your mind will not be at ease. So if your body can achieve what your mind desires it will be a body in a state of freedom and ease. On the other hand, if your body does not obey the mind it will be difficult to achieve the state of freedom and ease.

Q — Nowadays many people suffer from back ache. Is it difficult for them to achieve the state of bodily freedom and ease?

A — If you wanted to go abroad on holiday today but you could not lift things or raise your legs, your body would be impeding you so much that you would not be free and easy. So from this very simple example we can see that freedom and ease start with the body.

Q — Usually we are only aware of the body's existence when we are ill. We are only aware that our hands exist when they hurt. Can Bagua Daoyin enable us to be aware the body's existence?

A — Yes. Not only that, we will also be aware of the body to a finer degree. If our movements are coarse, then our mind will also be coarse; if our movements are fine, then our mind will be fine. Bagua Daoyin uses fine movements to train the mind to be fine. This is the first step to learning 'the unity of body and mind'.

Q — I understand that you followed your master for twenty-three years and were extremely close to him. Could you tell us something about your master?

A — Traditionally, becoming a disciple of a master was a mutual relationship of deep conviction. This is something that people today have great difficulty in understanding. However in the past it was a way of establishing a very close interpersonal relationship. I had this sort of relationship with my master, and my master with his master. When my master Gong Baozhai was young, he was sickly and was called 'coffin fodder' since people did not expect him to live for long. My master's uncle and my master's master, Gong Baotian, both worked in the palace, so my master was introduced to Gong Baotian to improve his health. From that time he was in and out of Gong Baotian's home just like a member of the family. In fact the relationship was closer than with his own family. This continued until he went out to make his own way in the world in his thirties.

Q — So was it the same for you, for the twenty three years that you were in and out of your master's home?

A — Yes. After I became a disciple my master's home became the same as my own. I went in and out freely, I ate there, slept there, mopped the floor, washed the dishes, put out the rubbish. This was all natural for the master–disciple relationship.

Q – This is certainly very difficult for people today to understand. Nowadays when you learn a skill, you have fixed hours of study and the relationship ends when studying is finished. If Bagua Quan cannot keep to this method of study, will it become a lost art?

A – This sort of study cannot be standardized and systemized. Unfortunately, to learn the real essence it is necessary to follow this method of living the life, what I call the osmosis style of study. With the evening class type of tuition of nowadays it is very difficult to pass on this sort of spirit. So if the heritage is to be passed on I recognise that we need to return to what I call the 'life for a life' form of teaching.

Q – If people nowadays are unable to receive this form of study, will not Bagua Quan slowly disappear?

A – I acknowledge that an art can disappear, but the truth contained within an art cannot disappear. When its time comes the truth will appear in another form. So what is important is not transmitting the art of Bagua Quan but passing on its spirit and attitude to life. If people today do not understand the 'passing on a life' way of living many things will fail to be passed on, which will create problems in people's lives and interpersonal relationships.

Q – This is an attitude towards responsibility in life. But people nowadays have a lot of complicated personal relationships. If they do not want to take on this sort of relationship can they still study Bagua Quan?

A – This sort of study is not a responsibility or a burden, it is a sort of guide to feelings and emotion. How can we study this sort of feeling? We first need to study our feelings towards our own body, to pay attention to it, to put this attention into our own body. This is the way forward.

Q – How can we begin to study to pay attention again to our own body?

A – As far as techniques go, Bagua Daoyin has some methods to guide you. Buddhism has a famous saying about life, 'during the time for eating – eat, during the time for sleeping – sleep'. Which means that whatever you do, put your whole mind into it.

Q – Is that the same as the Buddhist saying, 'life is for the present'?

A – Those who practice martial arts are the most likely to live for the present, since their life is on the line. The crisis and response are all in the present. Only if they handle the present well will they have a future.

Q – Although people nowadays have a complicated life and complicated interpersonal relationships, can they still master Bagua Daoyin and study how to 'live life in the present'?

A – On the first day of studying Bagua Daoyin, we practice putting your mind into the most basic movements. Life nowadays is very complicated but in fact it does not need to be so complicated. Returning your mind to the present is the first step.

Q – You have spent such a long time studying martial arts, and now you have put such a lot of mental effort into this book. Have you not thought about having some repayment in terms of fame and fortune for this effort?

A – If you use your martial arts training to seek fame and fortune the return on your investment will be very low. Just consider, it takes thirty years of training in a skill before you get a return. How stupid can that be? I remember my master used to say 'everyone wants fame and fortune, but let other people scramble for fame and fortune. True fame and fortune is what others give to you'. However since everyone wants fame and fortune, why would they give it to you? Because the more people you help, the more people will give you fame and fortune. So we only need to think about how to enable more people to gain benefit and not think about how to gain fame and fortune for ourselves.

Q – Bagua Quan is an ancient martial art. What do you think is its greatest benefit to people of today?

A – I earlier mentioned Bagua Quan's function of uniting body and mind. This is very important for people today, because society is becoming more and more complex, and changing faster and faster. If people do not know well their own body and mind, they can easily be torn apart by circumstances and will not become integrated people.

Q – What is an integrated person in terms of martial arts attainment?

A – Man only has physical and mental capabilities. So if we can successfully develop and control the abilities of the body and mind, we can be considered to be an integrated person.

Q – How in essence does Bagua Daoyin benefit the body and mind of people today?

A – Bagua Daoyin promotes harmony and balance in the body and mind. If you can attain this state of harmony and balance over the long term, not only will you have a healthy body and mind, you will also have a happy life.

CHAPTER 4

Paying for life with life – the master's apprentice years

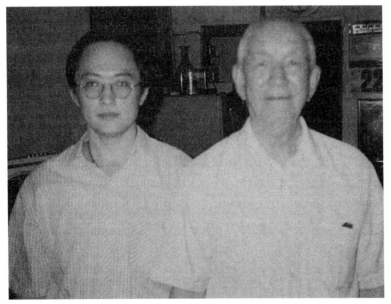

The author with the master

In 1979 when I was twenty-four I made the two most important decisions of my life – one was to get married, the other was to become a disciple to a master. Let me deal with how I became a disciple of master Gong Baozhai. At that time I was taking a course as a military serviceman at the Communications University and in my spare time taking part in the university's martial arts society. Through this I became acquainted with Professor Ni Weicheng of the applied mathematics faculty and through his recommendation I got to know Gong Baozhai. After a year of observation and tests the master finally accepted me as his disciple.

I remember that on the day I became his disciple the master wrote on a sheet of red paper the following 'the memorial tablet of the lineage of Bagua Quan masters'. He had provided an offering of fresh flowers and fruit on the dining table. The 74-year-old master knelt in worship and kowtowed before the memorial tablet to show that he was not himself taking a disciple but acting as the conduit transmitting the Bagua Quan pathway. Then we, master and disciple, in turn kowtowed to the memorial tablet and I kowtowed to the master. And so concluded the simple and stern ceremony of becoming a disciple to a master.

After the ceremony the master invited the memorial tablet to go outside, and burned it in sacrifice to heaven. This plume of clean smoke floating to the sky brought home to me the most important promise of my life. 'If you become a disciple to a master in the outdoors, a branch of a tree or a handful of yellow earth is then your memorial tablet. No matter what the form, devoutness is the most important factor', so my master instructed me in the unrestrained way of speaking of the Daoist school.

The connection of the family system is the blood relationship; the system of continuity from master to disciple is passing on culture. From this time on the master was better to me than to his own son and I made the master–disciple relationship and the master's teaching the most important thing in my life; to such an extent that I announced to my wife 'martial arts is first, writing is second, you are third'. And my wife graciously permitted my choice. For over twenty years every Saturday and Sunday was my martial arts training time. I am really grateful for my wife's understanding and cooperation.

My master not only taught me Bagua Quan he also concerned himself with my whole life – parents, children, work, the way I held my chopsticks – he corrected and instructed me in every way. Being a master is always a loss making business. The truth is that the master does not calculate the cost and spares no effort; he is responsible only for cultivation, not for harvest.

The master once asked me 'why do you want to practice Bagua Quan?'. I said 'because I like to'. It was many years later before I understood the meaning of that question. If we study to achieve some specific objective, when the objective is achieved the studying will stop. Only by following the Confucian maxim of 'doing nothing yet accomplishing everything' will you have eternal loyalty and really enjoy the process of studying. The master when he takes on a disciple must be quite careful. Over 20 years the master's disciples all went in different ways. Finally there was I at my master's side. I only then understood that the master's teaching was the 'osmosis' style. It had no set curriculum. It was a sort of accumulation of life – a contact here and there, some osmosis, feeding the dog, taking out the bird for a walk, playing chess, calligraphy, watching Chinese opera, doing odd jobs – all this was the medium of osmosis. My master once said to me 'the day will come when you will not know what you have understood'. Thinking about that now, do I really know what I have studied and what I have understood?

Is not the process of growing older like that? Imperceptibly growing older, imperceptibly enriching one's life, imperceptibly taking advantage of one's old age.

My life with my master proceeded like this for twenty-three years. Is the master–disciple relationship a teaching system? Thinking about it now I would rather say the master–disciple relationship is a sort of moulding of life.

However, what sort of skill and artistry is needed to succeed with this method of teaching? Since the culture can only continue if it is blended with the inheritor's life, this method of paying for life with life is indispensable.

Our everyday life cannot avoid overlapping with many other people's lives, but how many people dare make this mutual payment? How lucky I was in those two choices in 1979.

CHAPTER 5

Understanding Intuitively

There are some very strange coincidences in life which show us the way and help us to fulfill our aspirations. It is really moving.

When I was writing the third draft of this book, Jian Zhiyu of the Yuanshen Publishing House sent me a book on psychology which explored emotions and the mechanism of the brain and was entitled 'Love in the recesses of the brain'. This is an actual quotation from the book.

> 'The proper role which should be played by comprehension is to supplement the powers of recognition. It is as if, basically speaking, reason is a slow but sure method that a man who does not know the truth uses to discover the truth. Committing knowledge and skills to memory through feeling them is a way in which they will never be forgotten'

Good heavens! This was exactly the concept that I wanted to propose in my book.

The most important period of my studies with my master Gong Baozhai was when he was in his seventies and eighties. The things he taught me were mostly those he had studied up to the age of thirty – that is memories of fifty years previous. Usually if I asked him a question he would have absolutely nothing to say. But if I asked him the right question, or performed a movement that stimulated his interest, or he returned to the exercise area after practicing in his dreams, he would suddenly recall a mass of things that he himself had not realized he knew and reply to questions that you would have not thought possible to answer. This sort of knowledge that 'arises from emptiness' and 'seems to come at random' is often the most brilliant.

'Practice a thousand times, movements will be natural' is an old martial arts saying. Most traditional masters are not as talkative as mine. They will only tell you to train. Training is the solution to all problems. They consider that 'knowledge' comes from 'doing'. You practice and you learn, and when you know how, you practice some more. To have learnt and not to practice is equivalent to not to have learnt or even worse than not to have learnt.

Man's earliest knowledge was from observation. The Chinese concept of the human body is 'the heart is the repository of the spirit, the eyes see into the heart'. So the eyes are the windows that lead directly into the mind.

Traditional martial arts teaching follows this model. The pupil watches the master and practices by copying him. If his practice is not smooth enough, he watches again, tries to figure it out again and practices again. From studying forms to studying the spirit, from studying the outward appearance to studying the inner content, the key point is 'understanding intuitively'.

After language and writing became more explicit teaching tools and more important methods of teaching, the barrier between the sensory organs and the mind increased and communication between them decreased. Intelligence is like 'the presumptuous guest who takes over from his host'. Intuition has become underrated.

Consequently many people today have lost the ability to 'observe directly'. The brain is filled with knowledge, but the body doesn't want to act and try.

When a technique is lost, it can be recreated. When a 'method of know-how' is lost, the ability to create it is lost. What a loss this is, what a sorrow this is. We not only cannot learn how to 'unite nature and man', 'unite mind and matter', because we are thinking too much we cannot even make the proper choices and we are left in confusion. It results in our feeling slow and obtuse about our body and mind. What difference is there between that and being a 'walking corpse'?

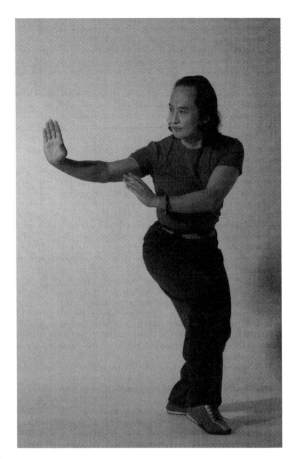

'See what is hidden behind what you see, learn the unknown through what you know' was the key for learning that my master used to teach me, and it is also the standard I have upheld for many years. Let us 'understand intuitively' and through this book begin to go back to learning through intuitive memory which will never be forgotten.

CHAPTER 6

Things you Ought
to Be Aware of when Exercising

   1. If you want to use methods of exercising to enhance your health, it is in fact very simple; you need only to: one – make sure that the exercise is correct; two – persevere.

2. Some exercises are designed for health (for example health drills) and some are not (for example all types of combat style exercises). If you are looking to enhance health it is best to clarify from the outset why the exercise has been designed, otherwise you will only achieve half the result with twice the effort and you may also injure your body.

3. There are two aims in taking exercise – keeping healthy and taking physical exercise. When exercising to keep healthy do it only until the body breaks into a slight sweat. In the case of physical exercise you must break though the body's endurance limit. Middle aged to older people should give priority to keeping healthy; there is no harm in younger people doing more physical exercise.

4. Before exercising you must warm up the body. Exercising that does not help the body to warm up should be avoided, for example stretching the muscles. Stretch only after the body has warmed up.

5. Unless you have a special training objective, do not exercise if you are too full, too hungry or too tired.

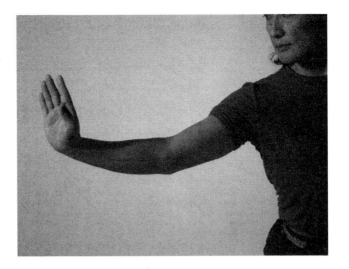

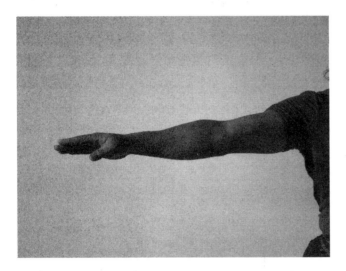

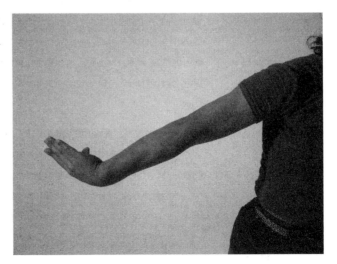

6. There is a saying 'avoiding the wind is like avoiding arrows'. While exercising and afterwards you must take care to 'avoid the wind'; this is especially the case in places like alleyways, corners of rooms, corridors and windows, where the wind is blustery and keen.

7. After exercising immediately mop up sweat or change into dry clothes. You must not let wet clothing stay on the body. It is easy to catch cold; it is better to keep the body warm and not get cold.

8. After exercising you should not immediately drink; you must wait until your breathing has returned to normal before drinking. Slowly sip the first glass of water and preferably drink lukewarm water; at all cost avoid drinking ice cold water otherwise it could result in the Qi circulating in the wrong direction and chronic blood statis.

9. After exercising you should not immediately wash in cold water but wait until the blood circulation has returned to normal, otherwise it could result in blood clots and even reverse flow which cause immediate damage the heart and micro arteries.

10. After exercising you should not immediately stop or sit down; walk around for a while without talking and let the body slowly return to normal.

11. While exercising you must be in a happy frame of mind; you should be able to quietly enjoy the exercise; you should not exercise when worry, depression and concern are at the forefront of your mind. This will not only negate the benefit of exercising but could have the opposite effect.

12. If you get real enjoyment out of your chosen exercise you will persevere with it. You should not exercise just for material benefits such as losing or putting on weight, putting on height, socializing or because it is fashionable. Only if you enjoy your exercise will it really help you.

CHAPTER 7

Give Me Fast Food, Nothing Else will Do – the Contemporary Concept of Health

Have you ever grown flowers? Have you ever raised pets? 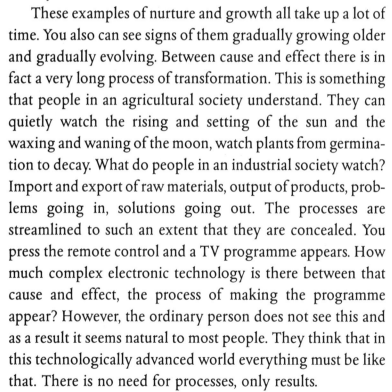 Have you ever taken care of children?

These examples of nurture and growth all take up a lot of time. You also can see signs of them gradually growing older and gradually evolving. Between cause and effect there is in fact a very long process of transformation. This is something that people in an agricultural society understand. They can quietly watch the rising and setting of the sun and the waxing and waning of the moon, watch plants from germination to decay. What do people in an industrial society watch? Import and export of raw materials, output of products, problems going in, solutions going out. The processes are streamlined to such an extent that they are concealed. You press the remote control and a TV programme appears. How much complex electronic technology is there between that cause and effect, the process of making the programme appear? However, the ordinary person does not see this and as a result it seems natural to most people. They think that in this technologically advanced world everything must be like that. There is no need for processes, only results.

Is it the same with health? If you have damaged some skin, how long does it take to get better? A damaged muscle or a broken bone needs over 100 days to heal. Cell mutation can turn into cancer, but many people in their pursuit of health want to be like mutating cells, switching immediately from abnormality to normality.

The majority of people are born healthy, otherwise they would not grow into adults. Healthiness is not comparative. You cannot divide up people into first and second class healthiness, or into physically robust and weak categories. Healthiness is the result of body and mind being in a state of balance. Anybody can lose their health if they lose this balance. People living today are tempted by so many stimulations. An individual's values, standards and position are under constant challenge. It is as if we were walking a high wire tightrope without a balancing pole. Those of us who understood our plight would be adjusting our balance all of the time. Those who did not think straight would be blundering on, gambling with their lives. However, human beings will go to stupid lengths to achieve their ends. Sickness and discomfort are signs from the body warning us to change pace. We must be careful over how we live in order to preserve our health. We must look after our health. Looking after your health takes thought and time. There is no immediate panacea, there are no quick fire methods. We must believe this before we can become really healthy.

CHAPTER 8

To Love Others you must first Love Yourself; to Love Yourself you must Love your Body

Is love a human instinct or an ability that is learned? If it is an instinct it will be something that everybody can do. Moreover, the outcome for everyone will be almost identical, just as when we eat to relieve hunger we feel full, when we put on clothes after feeling cold we feel warm. But it is obviously not so – different people can have different outcomes for their 'love'.

So does 'love' have to be learned – so that before it is learned a person cannot love? But how is it then that the love shown by small children can be more fearless and unconditional than that of adults? Either 'love' is really a human instinct, but one that has been forgotten by the present generation, or it has been distorted to such an extent that people living in big cities are unable to call on it or can only call on it with a feeble and frightened voice. If love is a forgotten instinct then it must still be in our bodies waiting to be brought forth. If love needs to be learned then who will be our teacher?

Is there anyone who because of love will follow us through thick and thin to the ends of our lives? There is only ourselves, there is only this body of ours.

Love is not a means, it is a feeling. Feeling is a way of delivering emotion – the subject of the delivery, the human body, needs to have the ability both to transmit and receive. If your mobile phone cannot transmit and receive a call or a message or its transmission and reception are inadequate, it is dysfunctional, no matter what its brand or model, how nice it looks, how sophisticated it is. If a person cannot correctly transmit and receive the message of love, they cannot be other than dysfunctional, no matter how attractive and graceful they are, how high their status, how accomplished their education.

Our body is a combined transmitter and receiver. To what degree of sensitivity can we detect the incoming messages and the messages within ourselves, or has the connection been completely broken? Are we aware of our own body? Can you sense your own body? Feelings of discomfort such as pain, aches and pins and needles are the body's way

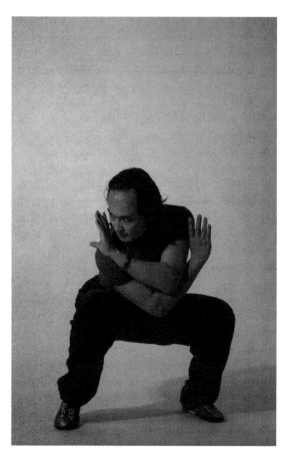

of making us notice it. Apart from this, are you aware of your body's existence? We often even ignore pain, aches and pins and needles. How often do we ignore the feelings of the people by our side – father and mother, husband and wife, son and daughter, our closest friends?

But why is this strange? If someone is incapable of feelings for even the closest 'body', if someone is in a 'shut down' state, that person is cut of from their emotions, basically not alive, a living corpse.

Do you want to become a fully alive person? Then first learn how to become aware of your body. Only when you have awareness will you show care. Only when awareness connects to the heart will you have love. You may think that you possess the whole world, but if you are not aware of the love between other people and yourself, then you in fact have nothing.

CHAPTER 9

Finding your Centre

The special characteristic of Bagua Daoyin is change. Why is change necessary? Usually it is because changes in the outside world affect our existence. We have no option but to secure the best foothold for ourselves while the outside world changes. The aim of martial arts is to seek survival. Is it not true that this is also the basic aim of everyone? In this rapidly changing multi-faceted world, each of us, no matter whether we want to or not, no matter how we try to hold out, is like someone who has fallen in to a raging torrent. We are swept along by the world around us. Will we be carried along, stupefied and panic stricken, or will we be the accomplished swimmer and take a grip on ourselves, mastering the flow and floating along calmly and gracefully until we can climb up the shore and look back over the water. Taking hold of your own centre is the precondition to mastering change.

Where is the centre of the body? Put your legs apart to the width of your shoulders, relax your knees, level your shoulders, sit square on your pelvis, pull in your jaw. Do you feel that your whole body is exerting itself without strain, but that you can stand as firm as a tree? Your head is positioned lightly in the middle of your shoulders, your shoulders are positioned lightly on top of your chest, your chest is positioned lightly on top of your waist, your pelvis lightly supports your waist and is positioned lightly above your

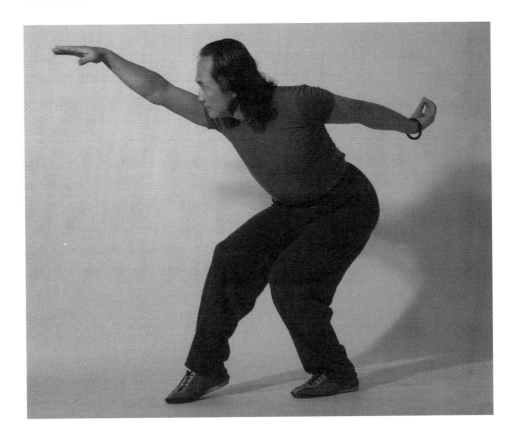

thighs, your thighs are lightly connected to your lower legs by your knees and are positioned lightly above your ankles.

There is now a wavering middle line between the body's stability and instability, running from the head to the pit of the stomach, the lower abdomen and the arches of the feet. This is the body's vertical centre line. Grasp this line, try to move it, try to use this centre line to walk.

There are two centre points on this centre line – the pit of the stomach is the body's centre point (that is from the head to the pelvis) – and the lower abdomen is the pelvic centre point (that is from the head to the feet). The abdomen in the front part of the body and the back in the rear part of the body form a cylinder between these two parts which is the middle region of the body. This cylinder is the middle region of the body. OK, you now know about the centre points, the centre line and the center region. Become aware of them, really become aware of their existence, grasp them, link them together. They are the keys that will enable you to change in a calm and unhurried way.

The pelvis is the body's base – it bears the weight of the upper body. Like the lower deck of a ship it has to maintain stability and balance. In fact the pelvis and the shoulders form two parallel lines across the spine. The level line uniting the two widest points on the pelvis is a middle level line. The intersection of this line with the middle vertical line is the middle point which provides a base for the body's stability. This is what traditional Chinese medicine calls 'huiyin' – the perineum position. Try to draw in this point of the body but without letting the muscles of the buttocks tense up (this needs a lot of practice). It is very beneficial.

The link between the body and the mind is a marvelous thing. Once you have established a centre for the body, you can set up a centre in thought and vitality for your entire person. When we have established our own centre we can grasp ourselves and find a foothold in this ever changing world, change in a calm and unhurried way and not lose ourselves.

CHAPTER 10

Opening up the Body's Unobstructed Space – a New Key to the Body

Is the body closed or open? Is the body solid, liquid or gas? Is the world in which we live closed or open? Is it solid, liquid or gas? 'The body is a small universe.' This universe is most definitely not closed. This universe is solid, liquid and gas simultaneously co-existing. The body is really the same as the universe. It is an open flow space and the flow within it is analogous to water and wind. In the body water is represented by blood and wind by Qi. So the body is a space in which the Qi and the blood flow. This is the key to the body being able to operate smoothly. However, there is a contradiction since the body is not a good space for flowing. Its small chest is packed full of things, the short limbs are divided up by three joints. It is extremely difficult for the Qi and the blood to flow easily in these circumstances. First of all we need to provide the greatest possible space within the limits allowed by the body structure, that is to open out the skeleton. We must pull open every joint which can be moved (such as the limbs) or cannot be moved (such as the breastbone). Normal postures must also be open and wide. If you hunch your back or spend your time slumped on a sofa, the Qi and the blood will be obstructed, the organs will not be supplied with enough Qi and the blood and will inevitably wither and become diseased. The Qi and the blood will

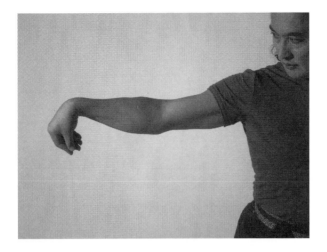

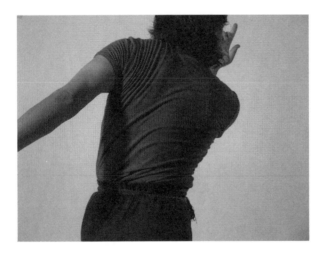

*Each joint has its own
unique range of movement
and method of movement.
We must clearly recognise
these and respect their
independence.*

decay if their circulation is obstructed for too long. This sort
of self-inflicted injury is commonplace in today's society.

Open up your joints, give your body unobstructed space,
give the Qi and the blood freedom to move – it is after all
your space and your freedom.

CHAPTER 11

Don't Use your Feet just to Walk – Teaching you to Make your Body as Light as a Swallow

It is very interesting. – man is born head first/feet last but dies from old age feet first/head last.

The feet support the whole of our body weight. A shop assistant stands for ten hours a day, a flight attendant stands from America to Asia, a ballet dancer performs on her points. Those enormous pressures are all withstood by those pairs of small and delicate feet. How can they put up with that!

After middle age an ordinary person often feels heaviness and tiredness in their feet. As time goes by the Qi and the blood cannot flow between the bottom and top parts of the body; they precipitate into a sediment and harden into immobility.

The legs and the arms are the body's limbs; the four limbs are like branches of a tree. They expand the trunk's living space but cutting them off adversely affects the trunk's existence. However if a branch is unhealthy it can infect the trunk and endanger the whole tree.

The hip joint unites the legs with the body and is the body's biggest joint. It has the body's largest muscle which connects the legs to the pelvic region and is an important source of life energy. This joint between the legs and body is a high precision design

However, during my more than ten years of teaching experience and in watching people walking about on the street,

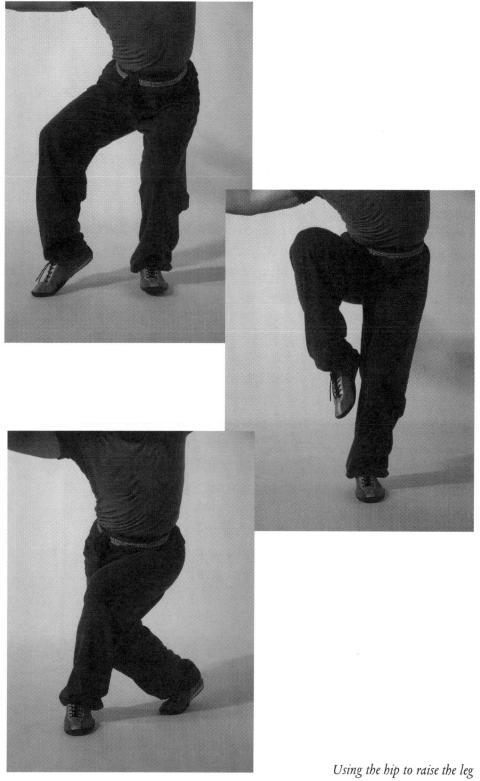

Using the hip to raise the leg

I see everyone walking and using their legs the way they have done all their lives but I have practically never seen anyone using their hip joints to walk. In fact many people do not even know that they have a hip joint to use – it is really hard to credit.

You cannot blame people. They have very few opportunities nowadays to use the hip joint. When you go into houses there are no high thresholds to step over; toilets are all now the sit down not the squat type; roads and paths are all smooth and level without any humps and depressions. So much so that physical demands on the body have greatly decreased and what you do not need you naturally do not use; and if you do not use it you find you cannot use it. However, the body's structure has not changed. The hip joint is still an important connection between the upper and lower body. If you neglect it, it will get angry with you.

Try using the hip joint to bring the upper leg back in the direction of the pelvis. Relax the knee and ankle and let them bend following the curve until the upper leg is fully raised. Keep the knee and the ankle relaxed and experience the comfortable feeling of the lower leg naturally falling under the force of gravity. Keep the knee and ankle relaxed and free and once again experience the feeling of the hip joint entering the pelvis. Gently shake and rotate the ball of the hip joint for a while then slowly move the kneecap from front to side and back again. Put the leg slowly down and raise it up again. If you can feel motion in the hip joint in each movement you will feel that your lower leg and foot are fulfilled and enriched. Congratulations. You have found your hip joint.

Try using the hip joint to lift your legs and walk. You should be able to feel that your legs are relaxed, that they are not an encumbrance on the body but have become a positive help. Slowly you will gain feeling in the lower pelvic area and the lower abdomen will feel enriched. Once again congratulations. You have started up your motor. Get ready to enjoy a new body. Yes, everything starts from the hip joint.

CHAPTER **12**

Relax, do not Collapse

Do you remember your most relaxing moment?

Taking a hot bath? Massage? Finishing a big exam? After love making? At that moment you didn't want to do anything, your mind was empty, your body was heavy, dissolved, enlarged, relaxed.

This sort of relaxation is admittedly very comfortable and benefits your body. However, how long can you remain in this condition? Can you carry over this condition to your life? If you cannot, then this is not the sort of relaxation that we want. It is called collapse.

Martial artists all know that they need to relax, especially practitioners of Taiji Quan. However there are very few people who can really relax. Some people who practice martial arts are saddled with a body of useless flesh and do not dare use any strength. Some people can scarcely raise a hand before their shoulders stiffen. This also is not true relaxation.

True relaxation must come from the mind and spirit. Only people completely at ease with themselves, fearless and undaunted, can completely relax. Therefore the human being is without doubt the animal which most easily gets nervous and tense. Isn't that so? You are afraid of not getting what you want. You are afraid of losing what you get. You are afraid of facing the future. As far as the past goes this was even more difficult for you. You worked diligently hoping that others would not look down on you. In every movement, every action, you were afraid of losing face.

Have you seen a carnivore hunt its prey? There are a lot of TV programmes which show this – tigers, lions or leopards using all their abilities to stalk their prey. But even if they fail they are still completely relaxed. They don't feel embarrassed. Other members of the pack, waiting on the side to collect an easy bald eagle or wolf, are not going to ridicule them.

Animals are relaxed all of the time. When they are systematically stalking their prey and you see their muscles sleekly rippling, this is the 'relaxing' that we are looking for.

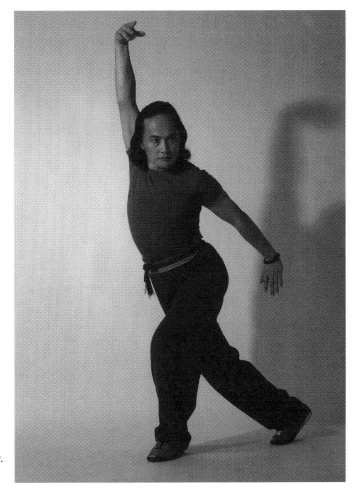

Relax before you stretch.
Don't stretch to relax.

True relaxation means relaxing the muscles. However, the bones of the body still have to provide a strong support. All movements use tendons to move the joints. Only under these circumstances can you relax with energy and gracefulness.

Bagua Quan requires you to

- 'Empty the centre of the palm' – not to grasp or grip or fasten onto things

- 'Empty the centre of the mind' – not thinking, pondering, or worrying

- 'Empty the centre of the foot' – putting the foot down to take root, lifting it and then walking, connecting the joints, relaxing the muscles, then completely relaxing mentally and physically so that you can perform free and unhindered movements and respond to life's challenge.

This is the aim of relaxing, this is the use of relaxing. If you collapse you have nothing.

CHAPTER 13

The Sexual Function is the Natural Manifestation of Bodily Health

It is said that over half of middle aged men are sexually dysfunctional and that many women are frigid, so to strengthen the sexual function aphrodisiacs are flooding medicine shops and the market. Medical specialists have made treatment of sexual dysfunctionality a separate branch of medicine. It seems that everyone has forgotten the original purpose of the sexual function.

Everyone of course knows that the sexual function in all animals is to reproduce the next generation. For this reason all animals have a mating season. For each individual Nature selects the most suitable circumstances to conceive and the sacred duty is instinctively performed when circumstances are best for the mating pair.

The human being it seems is the only animal that does not have a mating season. The human being is also the only animal that makes reproducing the next generation a by-product of sex. Sex as far as the human is concerned is recreation, social communication, self-confidence, conquest, trust, intimacy, attack, power etc, etc. However to see if sexual functionality is normal or not we must return to basics – the state of the body and the mind.

The sexual function is a natural manifestation of healthiness in body and mind since its objective is to produce healthy progeny. This outcome is the only healthy manifestation of the sexual function. Regarding the sexual function as just one of the functions of the body's organs and using medical treatment or external appliances to strengthen it is extremely dangerous.

The male sexual function consists of erection and ejaculation. If the penis is an 'instrument of exercise' this is the only type of exercise that does not use a muscle. The penis has a spongy tissue construction. After arousal blood flows into the spongy tissue so that erection and ejaculation can take place. The way that the penis works tells us that it cannot be exercised like a muscle. Muscle strengthening does not necessarily benefit erection and sometimes even has the opposite effect since a stiff muscle can adversely affect blood flow. The key to erection is in enabling the blood to flow freely. Therefore it is not surprising that warfarin, long used to treat heart disease, can be effective in erection problems.

A robust muscle needs increased nourishment from the blood so an overdeveloped muscle, in fact, produces an additional load on the body and inner organs. For example, the blood supply to the penis during sexual intercourse is relatively low. This is a case of something that is 'outwardly strong but inwardly weak', like a country that has built up its army and become involved in an unjust war to the detriment of its people's livelihood. This western style of 'health and beauty' should really be looked at anew.

The stiffening of muscles brought on by pressure can also adversely affect erection. Humans like other quadruped mammals contract their shoulders and buttocks when nervous. The original purpose of this reaction was to help us to run fast or to fight but for the person of today who gets nervous every ten minutes but has no need to run fast this has become a deadly instinctive reaction.

A small amount of alcohol can help with erection – not applied to the penis but drunk in a small glass before making love. In fact it does not aid erection but helps to relax muscles. Tenseness in the buttock muscles is the problem, so training muscles in the buttocks and the small of the back to relax can help sexual functionality. My male students often quietly ask me 'Teacher, can Bagua Quan help with this?' This sort of relaxation is in fact very effective.

The objective of sexual intercourse is ejaculation because only in this way can we reproduce the next generation. Semen is the essence that nourishes the body. It is like a perfume house which produces a few millilitres of essence by refining several tons of flower petals. It is an important key to the body's inner health. However the relation of semen to sexual functionality is in the timing and strength of the discharge. This involves the state of mind and muscular control. It is a complex matter which is best left to medical specialists.

The ideal process of sexual intercourse runs from the relaxation of foreplay to the gradual arousal of the body, culminating in the excitement of climax and then returning to complete flaccidity. Whether male or female, our bodily organs can naturally follow this rhythm. Using anything that interferes with this rhythm can damage the body.

The human being is perhaps the only animal that can enjoy sexual love. Make love by means of a healthy body and mind – do not just use the sexual organs.

CHAPTER 14

Menopause –
Grasp your Second Youth

 People have two periods of youthful vigour. The first is the stage of adolescent physiological changes, the onset of the development of male and female characteristics. The second comes after middle age; the female menopause results in the loss of child bearing capability; the male changes are not so obvious but can lead to a gradual decrease in sexual ability. Both sexes can experience physiological changes in what is called the 'menopause'.

We call the first period 'youthful vigour' and the second period the 'menopause' because we consider that the period from adolescence to middle age is a glorious stage of growth, that the physical and mental changes of adolescence are full of joy and hope. Even though the physical and mental problems of this period are greater than at the 'menopause', most people still have a more positive attitude towards them. The 'menopause' is regarded more negatively. We consider it to be a portent of old age and that old age is the threshold of death. So we are more pessimistic about the 'menopause' and even look on it as an illness.

I think that it is irrational to use these ageist values to label these two periods of physiological change as good and bad. We are accustomed to think that the human life span is seventy to eighty years, but is this true? There have been scientific reports that based on human physiology the proper human lifespan should be a hundred to a hundred and fifty years. People recorded in ancient Chinese texts, and Methuselah in the Old Testament lived for several centuries. If it is reasonable for humans to live for a hundred years the 'menopause' at fifty years is only halfway. Why should it be the boundary for old age and death?

My master Gong Baozhai lived to ninety-six. When he was over eighty he lost a tooth and grew a new one. This was witnessed by his disciples and members of his family. The master considered that at a minimum he could live to a hundred and twenty but later he progressively lost interest in life and became more and more estranged from the new era. In addition his wife died and the master departed after her. However he remained extremely vigorous right up to the time of his death.

The 'menopause' is a time for recovering youthful vigour. It is the start of another stage of life, a second youth. This stage marks a return to the period before adolescence where there is no great difference between males and females. Reproductive capacity again returns to zero in preparation for entering the second leg of the journey. The great pity is that our society gives its seal of approval to life values only in the years from 'youthful vigour' to the 'menopause'.

We do not understand much about the second period of 'youthful vigour'. If everyone considered that after the 'menopause' there was only old age and death, who would give any serious attention to managing this period of our lives?

If life is a circle, we usually only travel halfway around. It is like people in the past who thought that the horizon was the edge of the world. Nobody knew that another half of the world existed. From my master and from my body's messages I learnt the secret – that the 'menopause' is the second period of 'youthful vigour'. The days that follow are mellow and full of hope. Because we were able to use the first period of youthful vigour to set up family, establish businesses, take risks, make mistakes, study, grow up, the second period of youthful vigour can be for us a stage full of experience and knowledge. Can it really be that such a rich stage as this would mark the end of life? The female menopause is a positive message – it shows that life can take another direction and develop further. Let us drop this ageist standpoint. Don't pay attention to medical statistics. The world beyond the horizon awaits us. Life offers much more than this.

The internal organs are the body's soil – they supply all necessary nutrient to the body. Healthy organs are the basis for enjoying the second period of youthful vigour. Bagua Daoyin exercises go deep into the organs and strengthen them. It is from our personal experience in this that my master and I came to understand the second period of youthful vigour.

CHAPTER 15

Everything Comes from the Body – Entering Tranquility through Movement

Over its long history human civilization has developed many sciences, arts, religions and philosophies. Their discoveries and achievements have been multifarious and sometimes even contradictory. However one thing they have all found is that without attaining tranquility of mind, human beings cannot achieve their goals.

Tranquility of mind is the starting point for attaining any achievement. However, human achievements come at the expense of the tranquility of the mind. It is ironic. There is a stupid side to human behaviour. In the first half of life you put all your efforts into messing things up; in the second half of life you learn how to put things together again.

Tranquility of mind cannot be found directly in the mind because as the proverb says 'it is as unsettled as a capering monkey or a galloping horse'. The mind is basically a restless thing. Looking for calmness in it is as logical as doing what the proverb says – 'climbing a tree to catch a fish'. The mind is like a small child – restless by nature. However

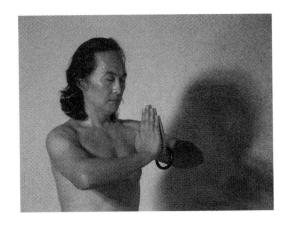

if a small child is engrossed by a toy it will calm down. Tranquility of mind is like this.

The mind depends on the body. If the body is not calm, the mind cannot be calm. For example, when you have toothache it is very difficult to be calm. According to legend, people who practiced Buddhism and Daoism to a profound level could transform things with their minds; that is to say if they had toothache and mentally told themselves that there was no pain, then the tooth would stop hurting. However, this sort of person is extremely rare. Before enlightenment even Buddha could not achieve tranquility of mind when he was hungry. From this we can see that when the body is not quiet and comfortable it is very difficult to achieve tranquility of mind.

To achieve tranquility of mind you cannot just ask the body to be still, because extreme calmness generates action – the more calm the body is, the more active the mind becomes. This can be seen when idle and bored people let their minds run riot and become afraid of their own shadows.

True calmness cannot be found by separating yourself from the world and seeking surroundings free from disturbance and pretence because the aim of tranquility of mind is to help us to live better. If like a monk you cut yourself off from society and look upon everything as of no concern to you, you will of course have tranquility of mind. However, that type of tranquility of mind is illusional. It belongs to the

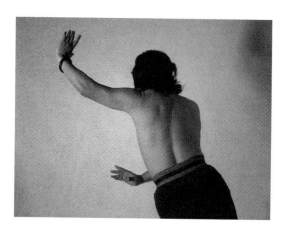

laboratory, it has not stood up to testing.

So for true tranquility of mind, you must first regulate your body and then train for calmness amidst movement, train for calmness amidst chaos, train for calmness amidst temptation, train for calmness amidst stimulation. Only then will you be able to achieve true, solid and beneficial tranquility of mind.

So let us start from this body of ours, which is closest and most intimate to us. When you have discovered the mind through the body, tranquility of mind will not be difficult.

CHAPTER **16**

The Song of Martial Arts –
the Form

The 'form' is rather like a melody in music or a sequence of steps in a dance. You can also compare it to the lyrics of songs and poems in literature. In my time as secretary of the Republic of China Martial Arts Association I saw that there was a great difference in what people within martial arts and people outside martial arts knew about martial arts. For example, we say that what Mr Zhang practices is Taiji Quan Paochui, what Mr Li practices is Shaolin Quan Paochui and what He Jinghan practices is Bagua Quan Paochui. The man in the street is not only unable to distinguish between these different types of Paochui, he cannot even tell the difference between Taiji Quan, Shaolin Quan and Bagua Quan. It is even more annoying that there are many people who take kickboxing sports such as Karate Do and TaeKwonDo to be the same as these.

Taiji Quan, Shaolin Quan, Bagua Quan, Karate and TaeKwonDo are classifications for different styles (paibie). They are also called branches (quanchong) or schools (menpai). They are as different from each other as classical, pop, folk and jazz are in the world of music. If you wanted to learn classical piano, your teacher could arrange a progressive course going from beginner through intermediate to advanced level. Every course has its model syllabus. For example, the Bagua Quan syllabus is on these lines:

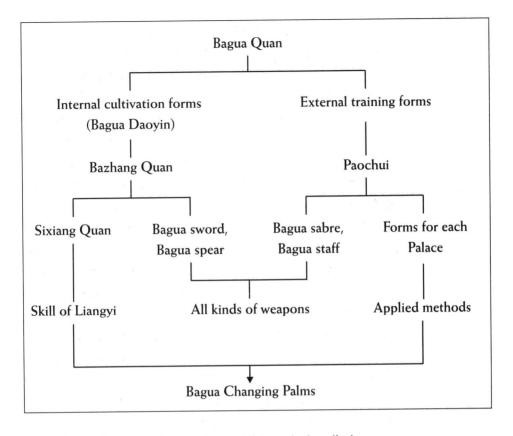

The above diagram shows that within a 'school' there are usually many 'forms'. This is the syllabus. If there is only one 'form', it is misleading to call it a school. Take Yang Family Taiji Quan. When it was set up, the founder put together a single 'form' to make it more accessible. It is as if the Italian tenor Pavorotti decided to make opera more accessible by teaching people to sing only 'Nessum Dorma'. There would be people who could only sing this aria. I know of students of calligraphy who practice by only copying Wang Xizhi's work 'Lanting Xu'. However, the aria 'Nessum Dorma' does not amount to the whole of opera. A single book does not amount to the whole of calligraphy. The transmitter of Yang Family Taiji Quan did not practice only a single 'form'. The 'public park style' and the 'adult education class style' are like the blind men sizing up an elephant and taking its trunk for the whole, or people looking at a leopard through a bamboo tube, getting used to what is wrong and mistaking it for what is right. It is a profound mistake for people to think that since Taiji Quan has only a single 'form' then Shaolin Quan and Bagua Quan therefore also only consist of a single 'form'.

As explained above practically all schools and styles of Chinese martial arts have 'forms'. The 'form' is a series of movements compiled according to a single aim or concept. The trainee practices by following the gradated sequence of the 'form'. It can be compared to a musical tune or a sequence of dance steps or the lyrics of songs and poems.

Many people, even traditional martial artists, consider that the 'form' is just a convenient way of remembering a sequence of movements. Others say that the 'form' is the way of extending the teaching session and that its purpose is to extract a greater tuition fee. This way of thinking is as ignorant as saying that the works of Shakespeare and 'Three Hundred Tang Dynasty Poems' are just a stringing together of ordinary phrases and expressions. I don't think that anyone would say that a melody is just a collection of notes. Of course in literature there are the 'Three Classics' and the 'Dictionary of One Hundred Family Names'. In music there are several teaching works of this nature which are simply for memorisation and practice. Martial arts 'forms' also have this sort of thing. Some music teachers say that once you understand about tune and musical theory you will be able to play any melody. However, nobody would because of this decry the value of all musical works.

Martial arts at their earliest stage indeed only consisted of isolated postures, just as in the early stages of language and writing there were only single sounds and single characters. The limb movements developed in the art of attack and defence evolved into a multitude of different 'forms'. They are unique to Chinese martial arts and could only have been created through the close amalgam of an age long history and a brilliant civilisation. This is a national asset which is underdeveloped since the Chinese people do not yet fully understand it.

Every traditional 'form' has an aim. Some aim to explain in a succinct way the core contents of a martial arts style. Some aim to practice a certain skill. Some aim to correct a posture or embed a routine. Some aim to demonstrate the application of change and development. Some are as long as two hundred or three hundred movements, some have only ten or twenty postures. However, no matter what, a good 'form' will be rationally composed from beginning to end, that is to say all stages of the movements in the 'form' will correspond with the rhythm of breathing and the smoothness of the movement of the limbs. Otherwise it could lead to obstruction of the Qi and the blood. This goes against the aim of practicing martial arts. No master would ruin his disciple in this way unless his disciple were training to become a killer.

We can imagine the 'form' as a song without words because every 'form' has its own special metre and rhythm. We can imagine it as a dance because it has its own special language of the limbs. We can regard it as a work of literature because of what its contents relate to us. Looking at the 'form' in this way we can see the wisdom and intent of our forebears. We will surely be convinced that the culture passed on through time and space by so many generations worth of personal verification must have diamond like quality.

CHAPTER 17

Shape, Potential Force and Spirit in Posture

The greatest difference between movement in martial arts and dance steps or physical training is that the effort generated by martial arts movement has a clear aim and direction. Movement produces the basic elements of shape (xing), potential force (shi) and spirit (shen).

The first step in practicing any martial arts style is to open up the body's skeleton. This is the stage of 'correcting the body' which will allow the trainee to open the joints, correct the posture and establish a body structure matching the requirements of the specific martial arts style. Only when this has been achieved can the shapes and patterns of posture changes be copied. So at this stage, regular teaching programs in all styles and schools include much polishing and refinement.

'Shape' in martial arts has just two objectives. One is to resist the external enemy. The other is to cultivate the inner body. Concentrating on the second objective is what is denoted by 'intent' (yi). This brings 'spirit', guides 'shape' and produces 'potential force'.

A movement in martial arts is bound to have 'potential force'. 'Potential force' can be found in the power generated by the switch between action and rest. A tiger lying in the sun has 'shape' without 'potential force' – but if it lies on its belly making 'potential force' ready to leap, then there is force concealed within.

If the limbs can produce a correct movement in response to needs, the line of intent of the 'spirit' can lead to a correct 'shape'. Within a correct 'shape' there is a correct flow of Qi and blood. This produces the 'potential force' required to produce the posture. These three essential factors complement each other, and for the successful martial artist all stable and well balanced standing and sitting postures are like this.

So 'shape', 'potential force' and 'spirit' are not just the prerogatives of the martial artist; they should be naturally present in any person who is sound in mind and body and has a good energy level. We can see a great difference in 'shape', 'potential force' and 'spirit' between a vigorous energetic person and someone who is listless and dejected. Practicing martial arts is the best way for us to establish 'shape', 'potential force' and 'spirit'. This is also the most important aspect of martial arts for people today.

Bagua Daoyin concentrates on this approach to build up and foster awareness and practice of 'shape', 'potential force' and 'spirit'.

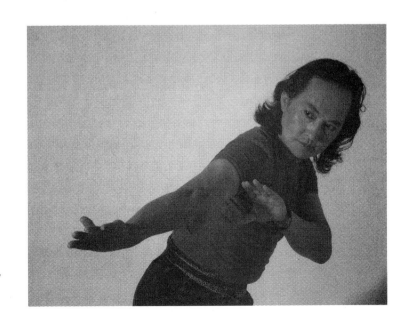

Through the fingertips guide the pathway prepared by the shape, potential force and spirit

CHAPTER 18

Between Yin and Yang

Chinese culture is the culture of Yin and Yang. This is something everyone knows. However, there are differing explanations about the meaning of Yin and Yang. Many people reckon that Yin and Yang are concepts which are opposed and contradictory. However such an explanation of Chinese culture is incorrect as far as we practitioners of Bagua Quan are concerned. Yin and Yang in themselves are of course opposites, so we use Yin and Yang to generalise opposing elements such as up and down, left and right, day and night, water and fire, male and female, inside and outside. But Yin and Yang do not exist in separated and independent forms. Yin and Yang are two faces of a whole, or, it may be said, Yin and Yang join together and combine into a whole.

A circle has 360 degrees and so from the centre of a circle to its circumference there are 360 divisions. Yin and Yang are two divisions called 'Liangyi' (literally: two rituals). If the Liangyi flow, grow and decline in a clockwise direction, that is to say if to start with Yang is on the left side and Yin on the right side, their position will be balanced and they may produce a transitional stage, the Sixiang (literally: four images), which is also the four quadrants of a circle. In this instance it is not enough to use the two words Yin and Yang. The original Yin should be called 'YinYin' and the original

Yang 'YangYang'. The transitional area between YinYin and YangYang is called 'YinYang' and the transitional area between YangYang and YinYin is called 'YangYin'. These are the respective names of the Sixiang. From this it follows that the Bagua (eight trigrams), or eight division circle, is composed of three Yin Yang symbols and the Liushigegua (sixty-four trigrams) are composed of six Yin Yang symbols.

CHAPTER 19

Sixiang Quan

 The fundamental Bagua Quan Yin and Yang changes are based on the Sixiang

- YangYang (greater Yang) changes YangYin (lesser Yin)

- YangYin changes YinYin (greater Yin) or YinYang (lesser Yang)

- YinYin changes YinYang

- YinYang changes YangYang or YangYin.

○ YangYang indicates the part of the body and direction of movement above the shoulders (called the upper pathway).

○ YinYin indicates the part of the body and movements below the stomach (called the lower pathway).

○ YangYin indicated centre movements with changes from above to below, usually between the chest and the stomach (called the centre pathway).

○ YinYang indicates centre movements with changes from below to above (belonging to the centre pathway).

Because YinYang and YangYin relate to the left and right of the centre pathway they can interchange.

These are the foundation principles for change in Bagua Quan and can lead you to a deeper understanding.

In the complete system of Bagua Quan the following four postures are used to represent the Sixiang:

Golden cockerel standing on one leg (YangYang)

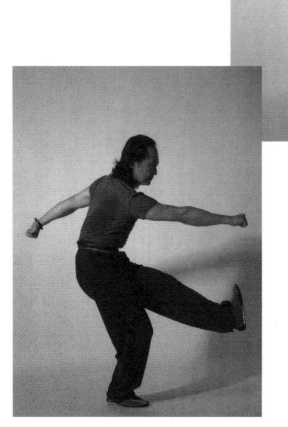

Cross punch (shizi chui) (YangYin)

Magpie alights on a branch (YinYang)

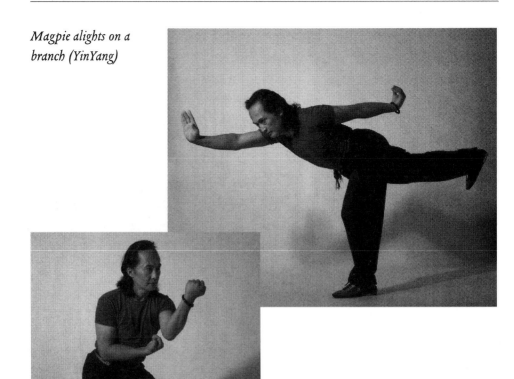

Phoenix circles over its nest (YinYin)

The development and linking together of these four postures produce Sixiang Quan.

In the Yin and Yang Bagua system, 'Liangyi' has life without shape and pattern, while 'Sixiang' has shape and pattern without life. Each shape and pattern in the 'Sixiang' attains the two Yin and Yang lives of 'Liangyi' and becomes the all encompassing 'Bagua'. The 'Sixiang' in the human body indicate the four limbs. Sixiang Quan movements have the purpose of training the four limbs.

The root of the arms is in the shoulder blades. The root of the legs is in the knee joints. Above and below these unite in the waist. The movements of Sixiang Quan seek to put to use the roots of the four limbs.

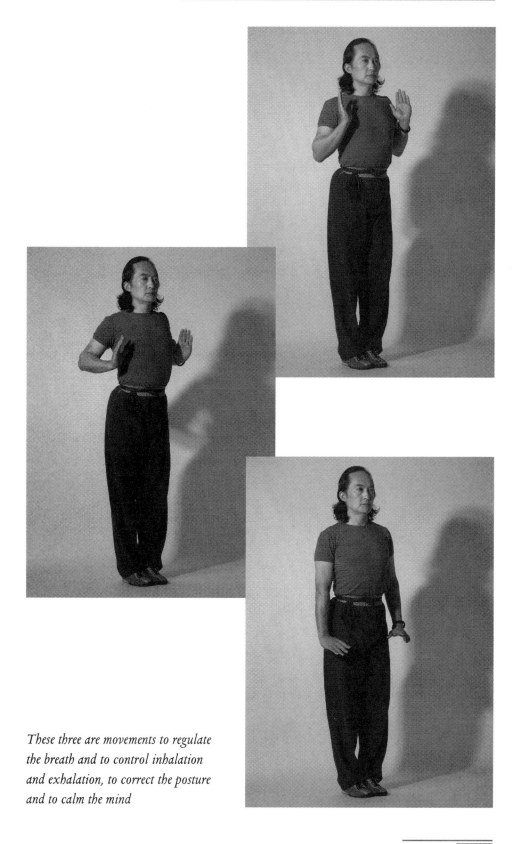

*These three are movements to regulate
the breath and to control inhalation
and exhalation, to correct the posture
and to calm the mind*

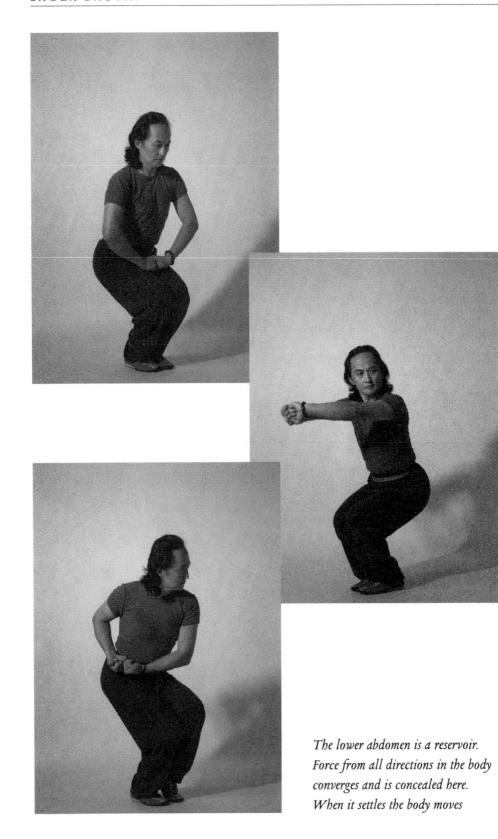

The lower abdomen is a reservoir.
Force from all directions in the body
converges and is concealed here.
When it settles the body moves

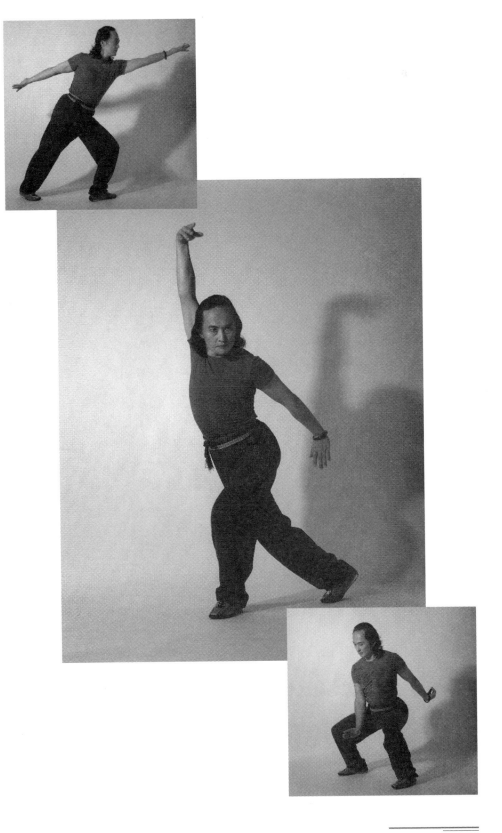

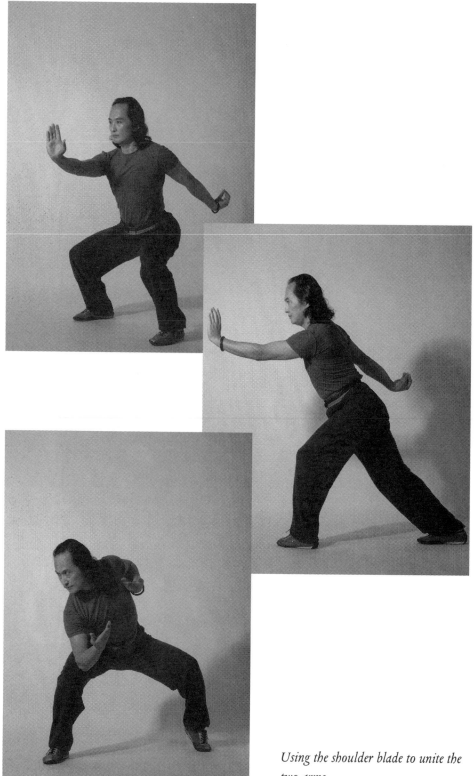

Using the shoulder blade to unite the two arms

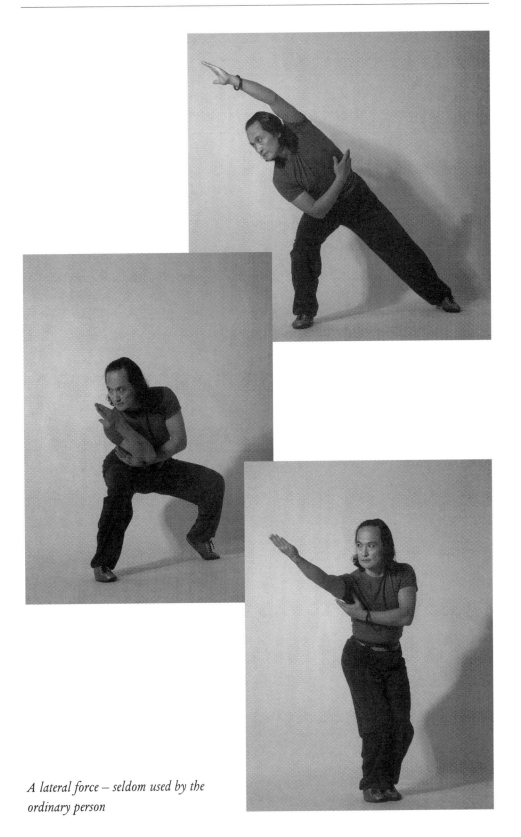

*A lateral force – seldom used by the
ordinary person*

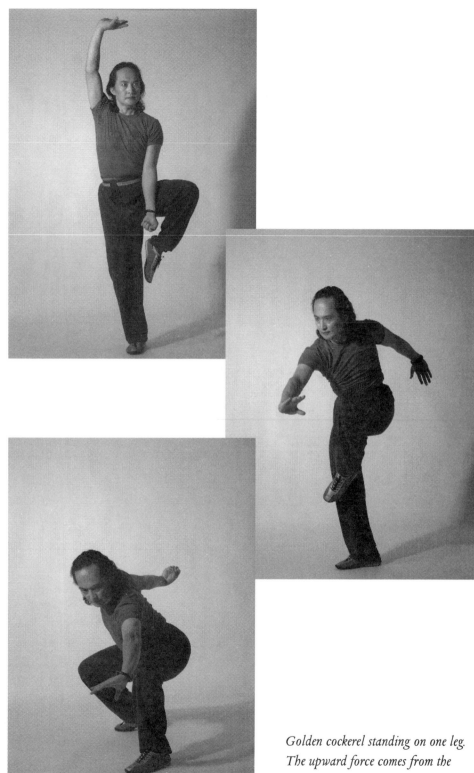

*Golden cockerel standing on one leg.
The upward force comes from the
downward counterforce*

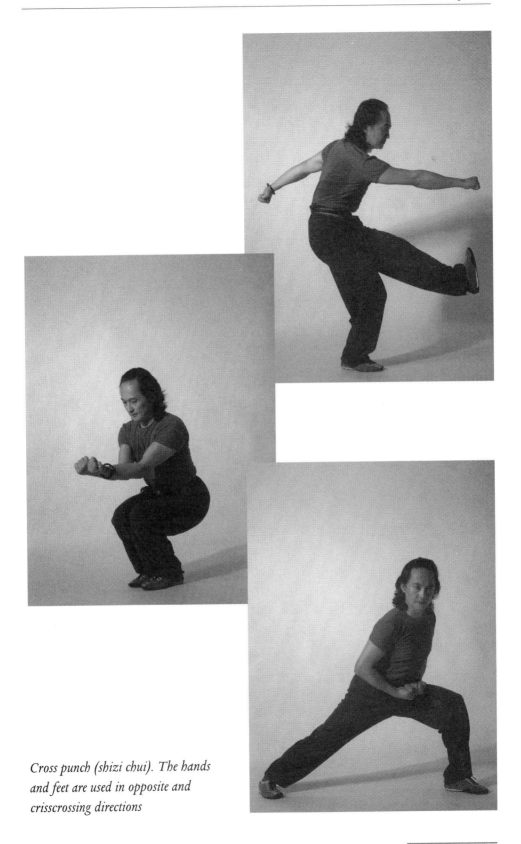

Cross punch (shizi chui). The hands and feet are used in opposite and crisscrossing directions

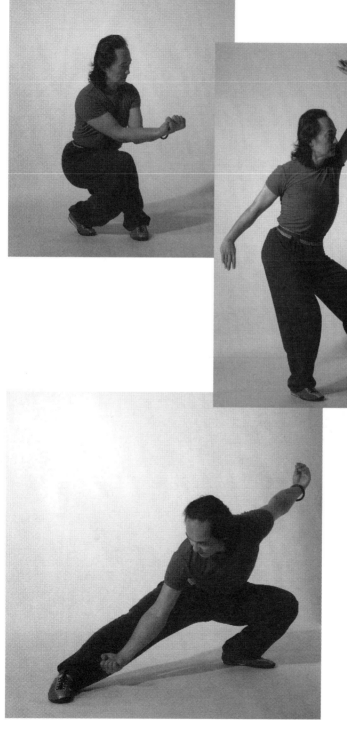

Revolving punch (xuan chui)

*Returning body punch
(fanshen chui)*

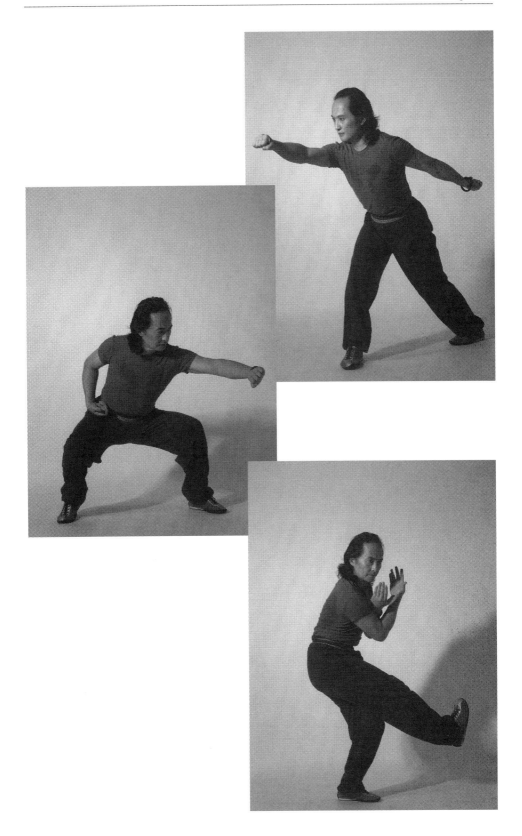

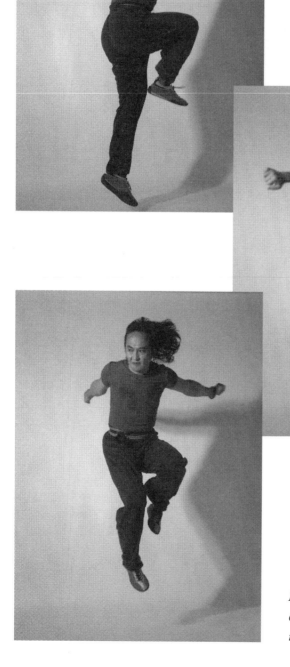

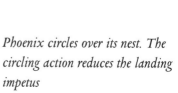

Phoenix circles over its nest. The circling action reduces the landing impetus

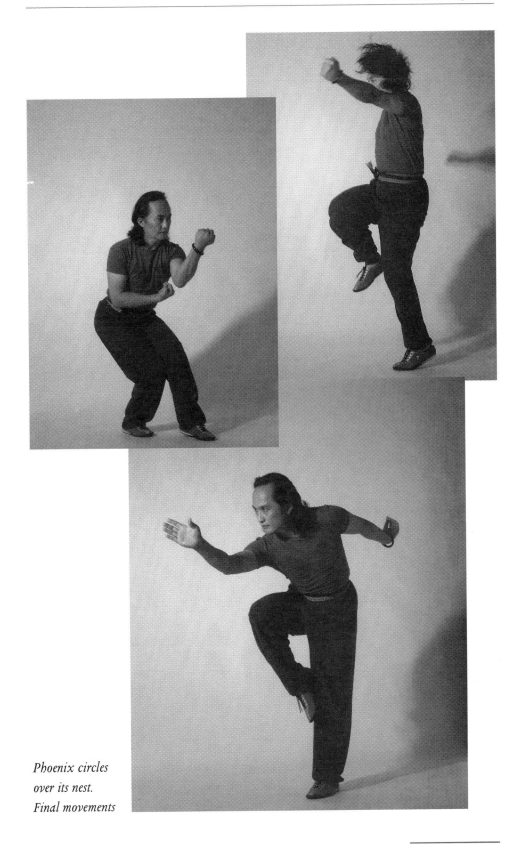

*Phoenix circles
over its nest.
Final movements*

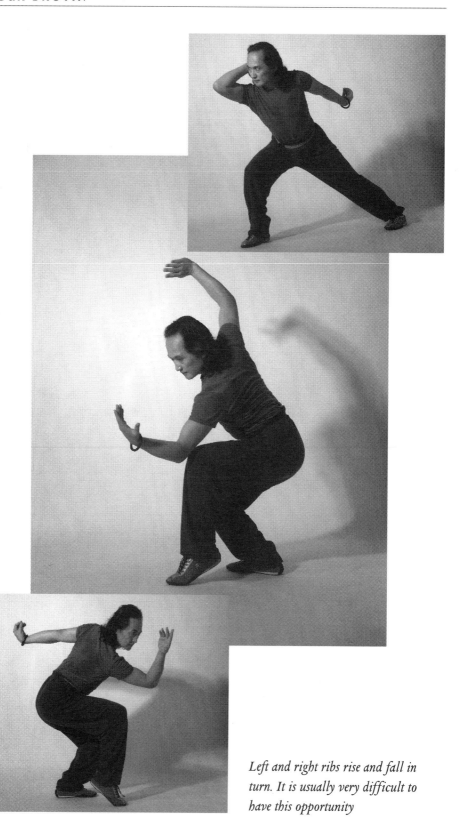

Left and right ribs rise and fall in turn. It is usually very difficult to have this opportunity

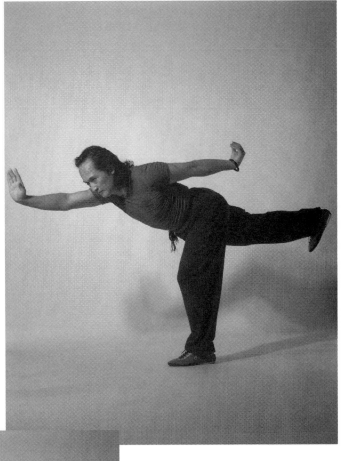

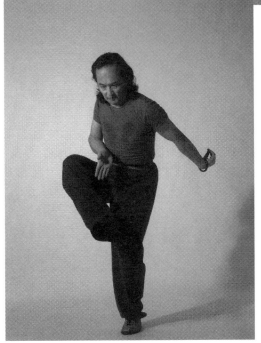

Magpie alights on a branch

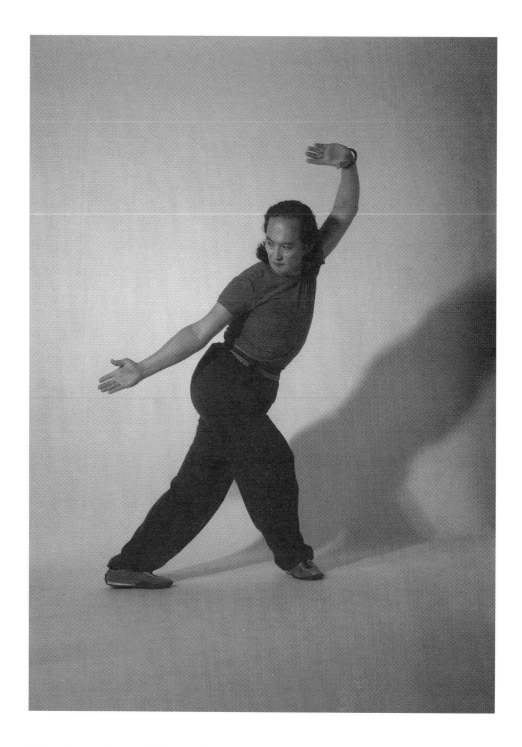

The twist turn is a special feature of Daoyin

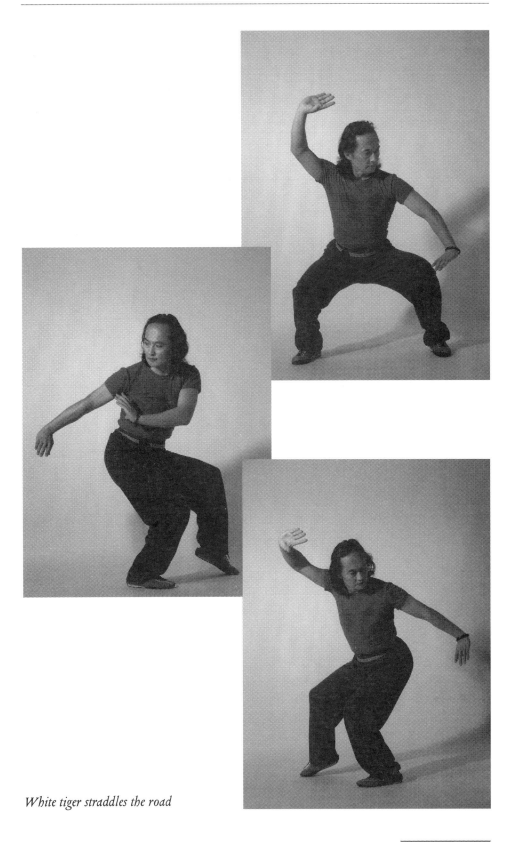

White tiger straddles the road

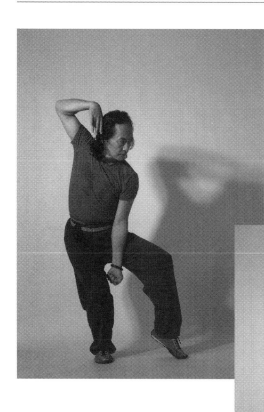

The right elbow is raised and the left elbow falls. The body feels great

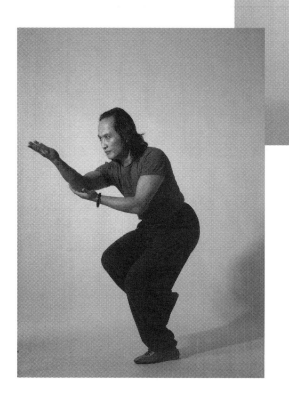

Chilin spits out the book

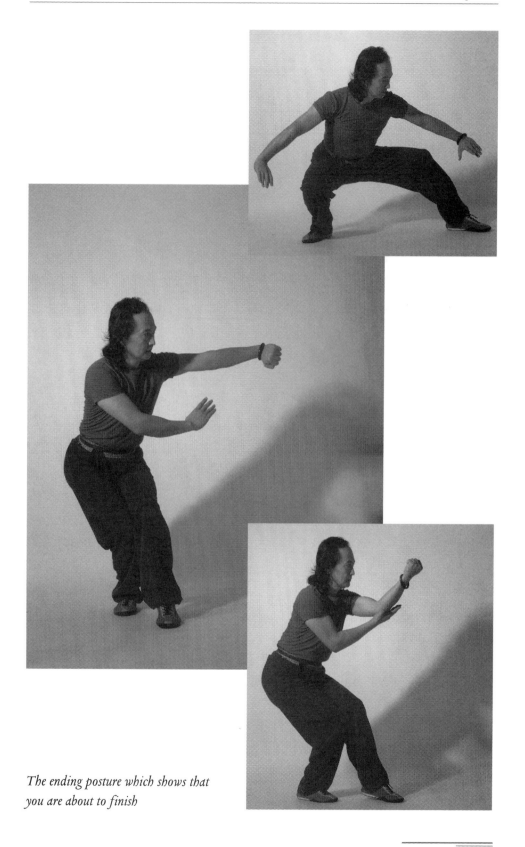

The ending posture which shows that you are about to finish

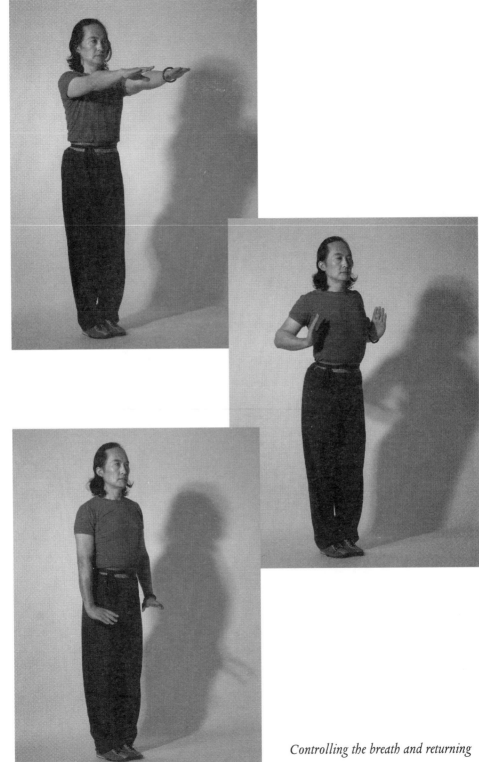

*Controlling the breath and returning
to the start position*

CHAPTER 20

The Melody of the Flow – Bazhang Quan

At the heart of Bagua Quan there are eight basic postures that are called 'Eight Mother Palms' (bamuzhang). These eight postures display eight palms in a static state; each palm individually stands alone and does not inter-relate to the others.

Although the Eight Mother Palms are eight palms postures, it is in fact the Bagua (eight trigrams) which assume the two Yin and Yang aspects of the Sixiang (four images).

- 'Red phoenix faces the sun' is the Yin side of YangYang (internally associated with the heart)

- 'Lion opens wide its mouth' is the Yang side of YangYang (externally associated with the head)

- 'White ape offers fruit' is the Yin side of YangYin (internally associated with the lung)

- 'Black tiger comes out from the cave' is the Yang side of YangYin (externally associated with the back)

- 'White snake slithers through the grass' is the Yin side of YinYin (internally associated with he kidney)

- 'Chilin spits out the book' is the Yang side of YinYin (externally associated with the abdomen)

- 'Green dragon flies upwards' is the Yin side of YinYang (internally associated with the liver)

- 'Great roc spreads its wings' is the Yang side of YinYang (externally associated with the waist/lower back)

Therefore the changes in the eight palms can be induced through the Yin and Yang changes of the Sixiang. Bazhang Quan (eight palms martial arts style) is consequently a first rate model.

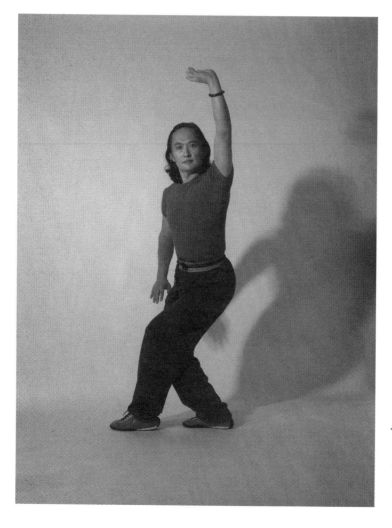

1. Red phoenix faces the sun (leads to a strengthening of the heart - Yang Yang)

2. *White ape offers fruit (leads to a strengthening of the lungs – Yang Yin)*

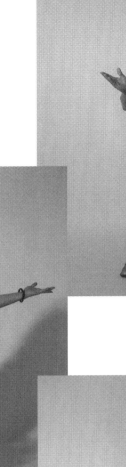

3. *Green dragon flies upwards (leads to a strengthening of the liver – YinYang)*

4. *White snake slithers through the grass (leads to a strengthening of the kidneys – YinYin)*

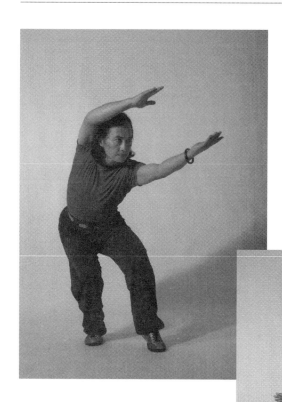

5. Lion opens wide its mouth (suitable for the head – Yang Yang)

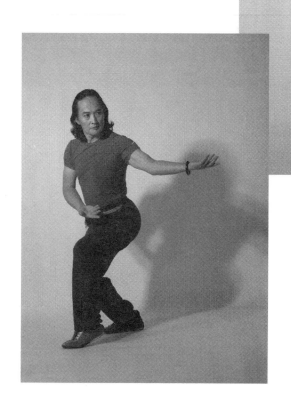

6. Black tiger comes out of the cave (helps to link up shoulders and back – Yang Yin)

7. Great roc spreads its wings (stretches and strengthens the waist / lower back – Yin Yang)

Bazhang Quan has Eight Mother Palms as its backbone. It is constructed by taking 'static eight palms' and, in accordance with the principles of Yin and Yang, linking them together through moves and changing them into 'dynamic eight palms'. An inter-relationship is thereby created between the eight palms. It is as if eight singers came together in a chorus.

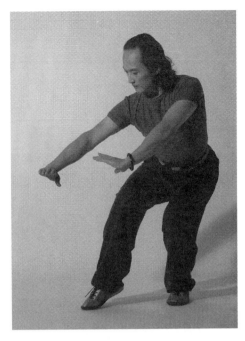

8. Chilin spits out the book (calms and strengthens the abdomen – Yin Yin)

'Dynamic eight palms' and 'static eight palms' have entirely different shapes and appearance. It is like the difference in appearance between a silent, unsmiling person and somebody who is talking and laughing cheerfully. Nevertheless they are basically the same inside.

The most important aspect of 'static eight palms' is to practice using external force to direct inner Qi and thereby achieve the aim of 'combining inner Qi and movement'. This means through static exercises gaining an understanding of the relationship between the postures and the inner organs, the meridians, Qi and blood.

When we have acquired this feeling and ability we can learn how to apply 'dynamic Bazhang Quan' to use inner Qi to drive external force. This means operating Qi and blood and the meridians within the body to regulate and control the body and mind. Therefore in the Bagua Quan system this is the leading form for internal cultivation work.

The significance of Bazhang Quan does not consist in just exercising single movements but in providing a complete understanding of the principles of flow and change between the eight palms and of the proper order of exercise of the eight palms of Bazhang Quan.

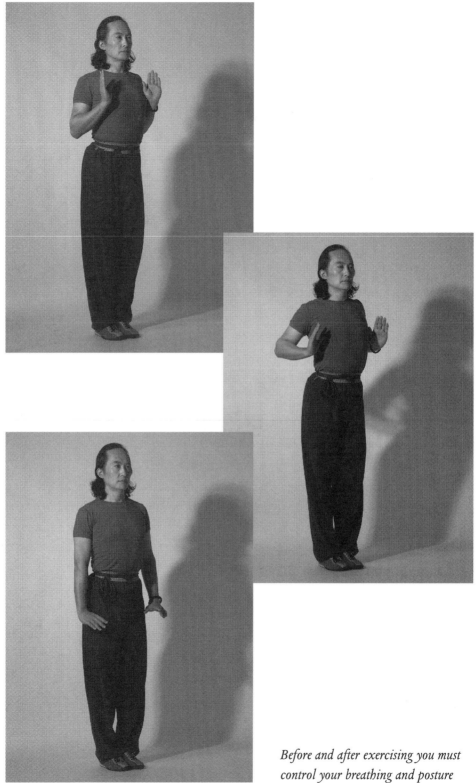

Before and after exercising you must control your breathing and posture

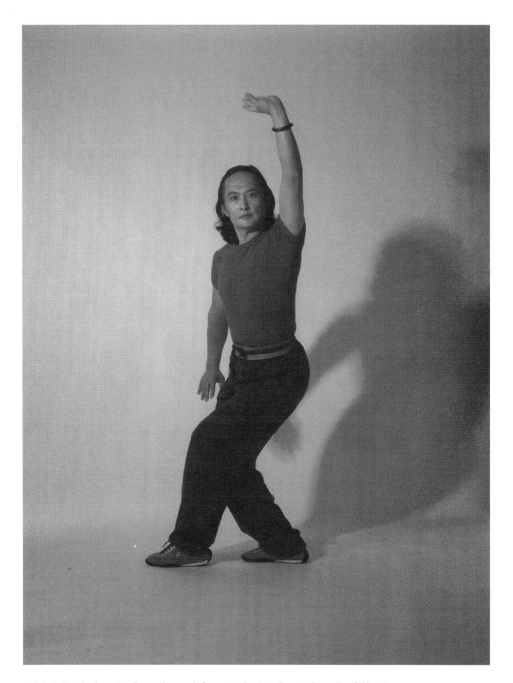

This is 'Red phoenix faces the sun' from Eight Mother Palms; the following movements are derived from it

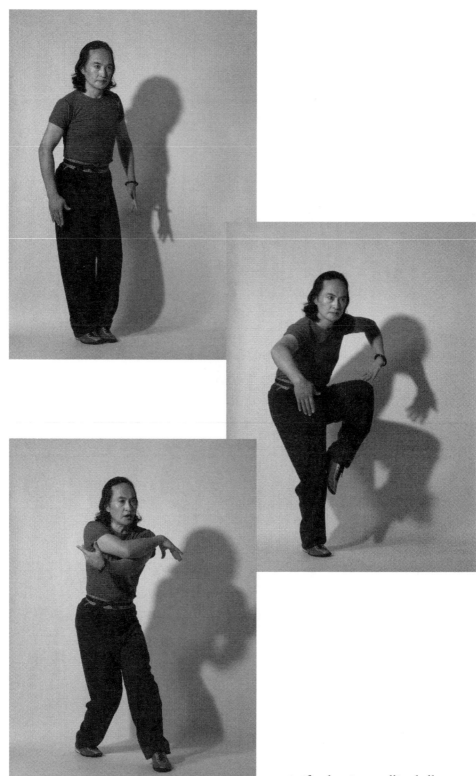

As if embracing a rolling ball

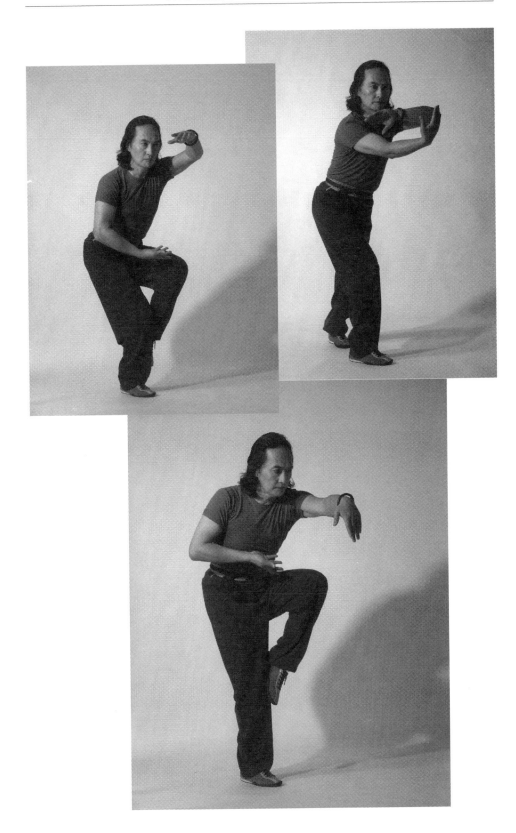

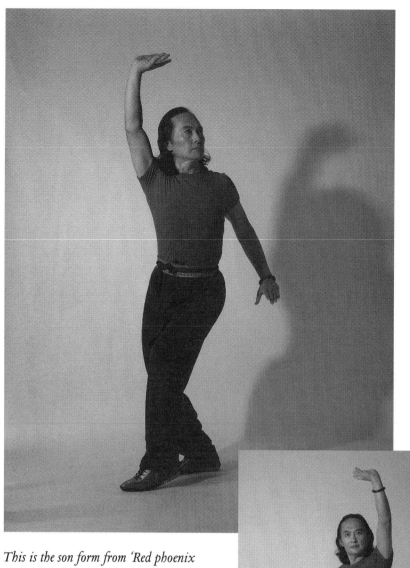

This is the son form from 'Red phoenix faces the sun'

This is the mother form

This is 'Black tiger comes out from the cave' from Eight Mother Palms; the movements below are derived from it

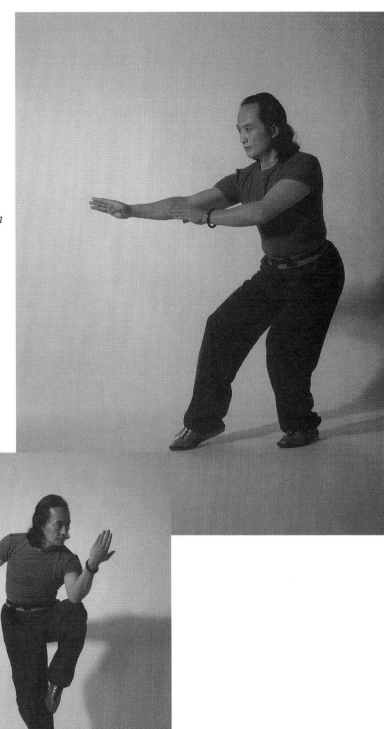

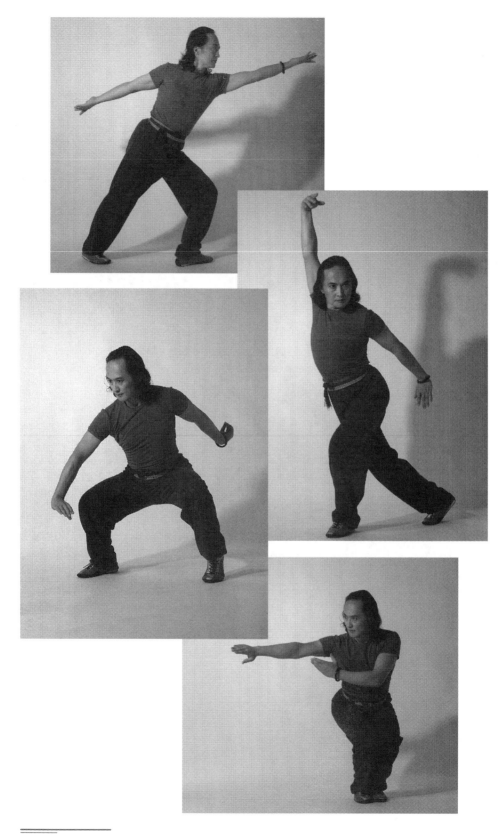

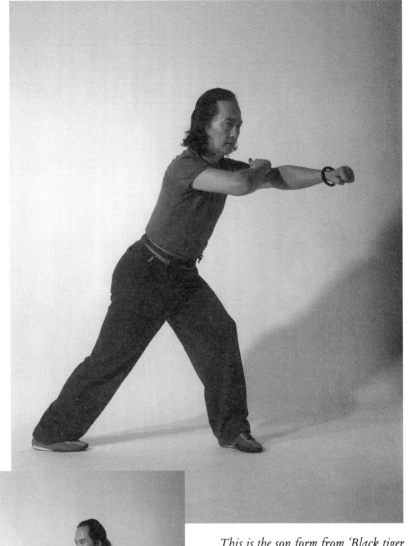

*This is the son form from 'Black tiger
comes out from the cave'*

This is the mother form

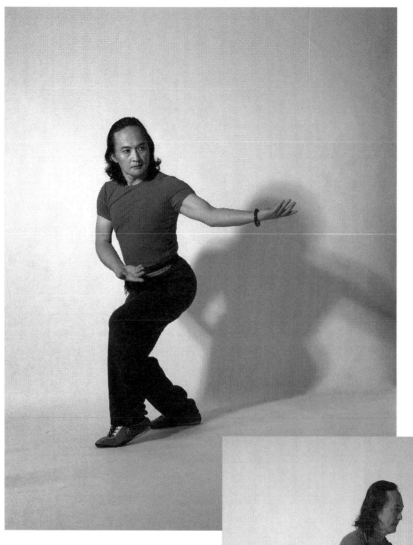

*This is 'Great roc spreads its wings'
from Eight Mother Palms; the
following*

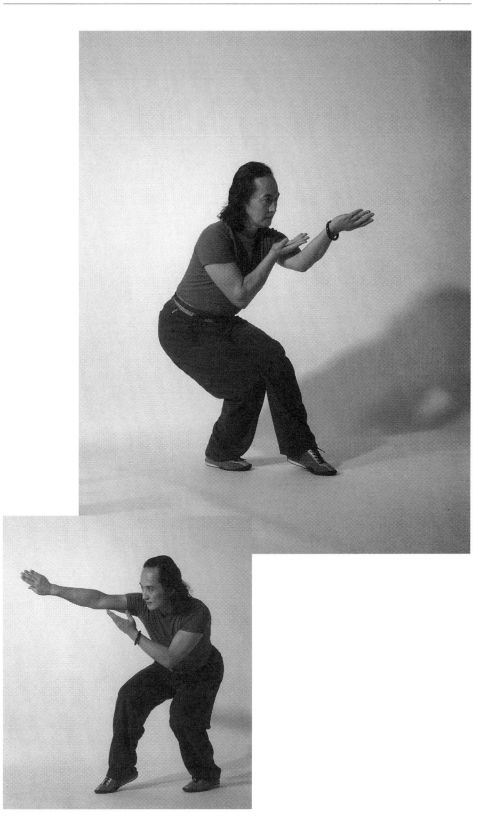

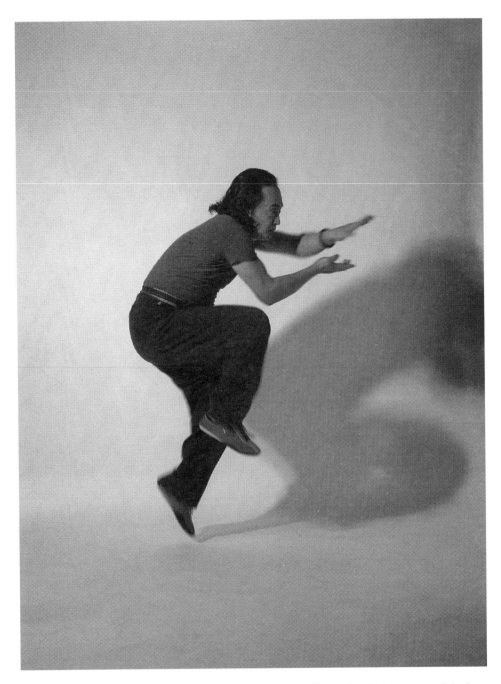

Contracting the body to change step; the hip joint must be able to absorb the impact of the legs

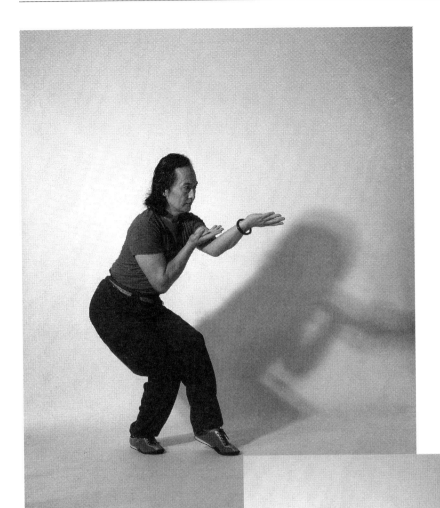

This is the son form from 'Great roc spreads its wings' movements are derived from it

This is the mother form

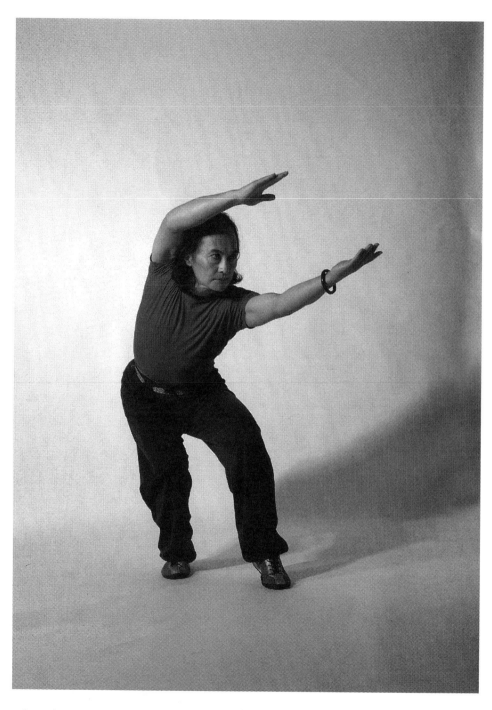

This is 'Lion opens wide its mouth' from Eight Mother Palms; the following movements are derived from it

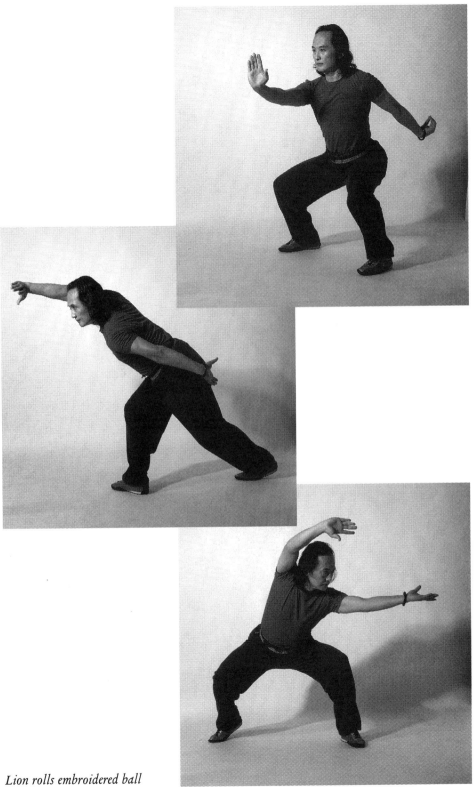

Lion rolls embroidered ball

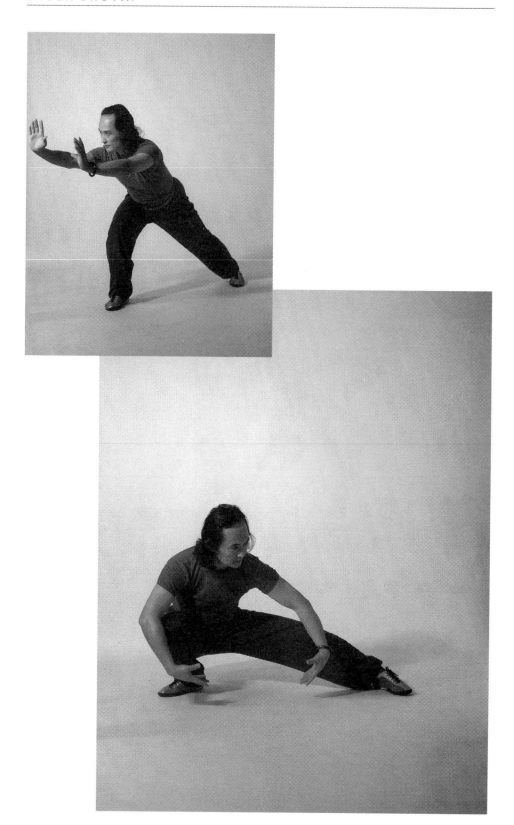

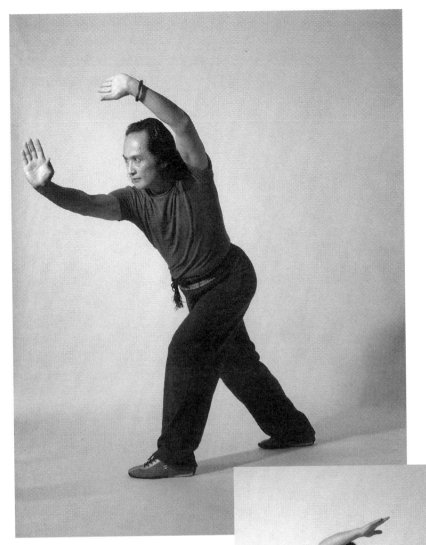

This is the son form from 'Lion opens wide its mouth'

This is the mother form

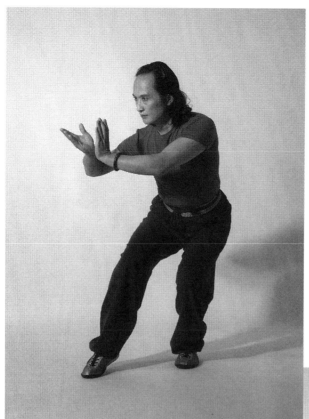

This is 'White ape offers fruit' from Eight Mother Palms; the following movements are derived from it

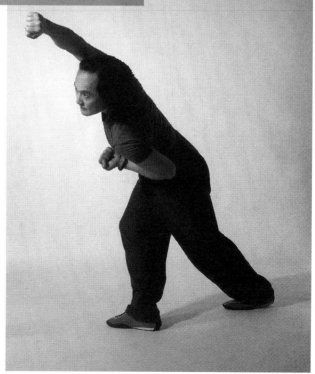

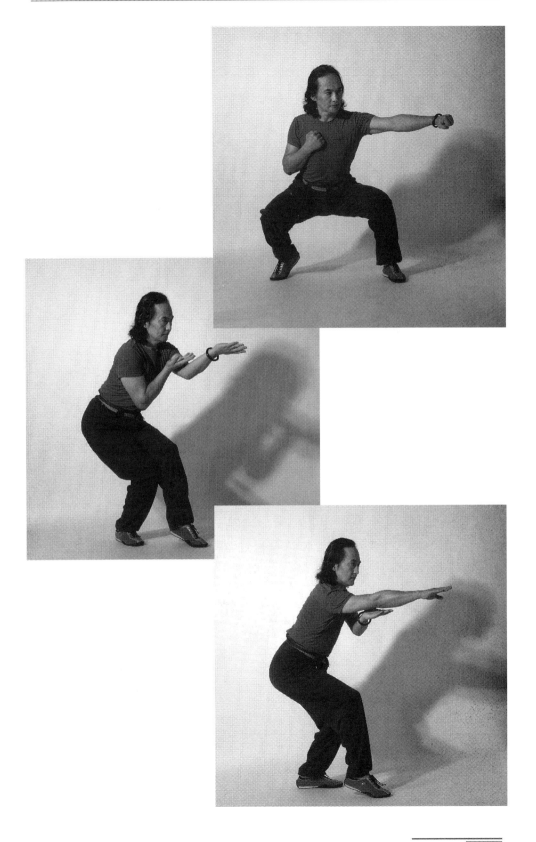

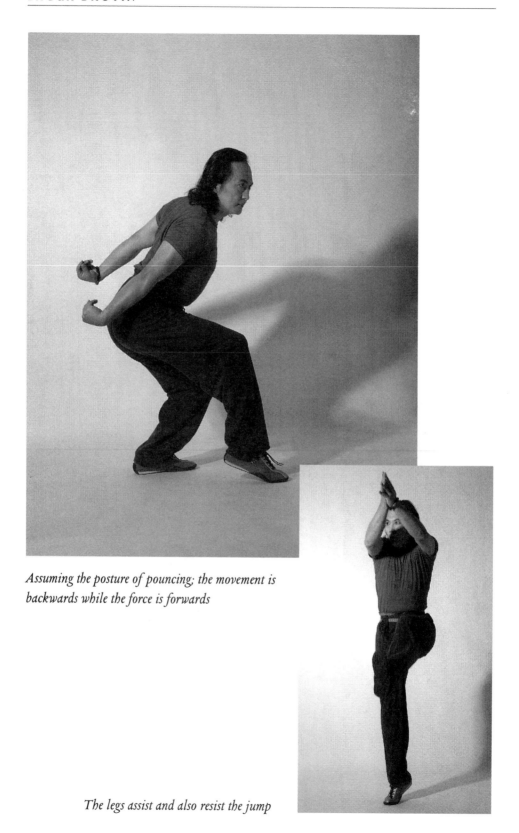

*Assuming the posture of pouncing; the movement is
backwards while the force is forwards*

The legs assist and also resist the jump

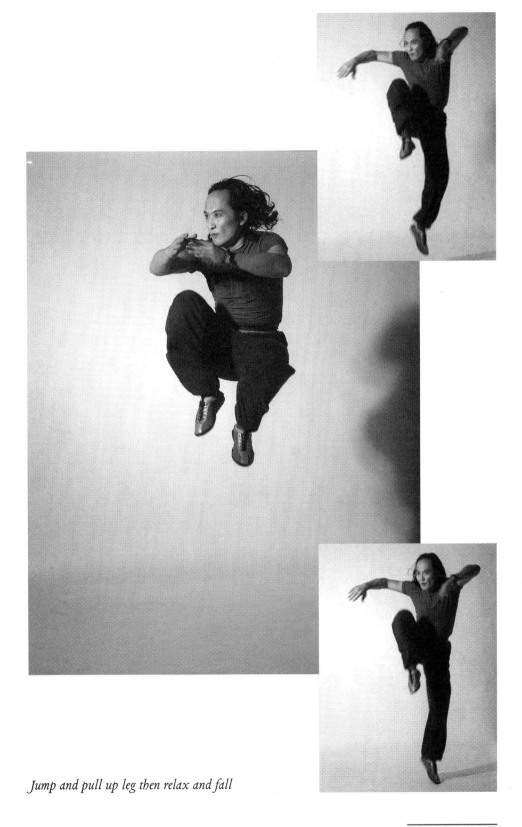

Jump and pull up leg then relax and fall

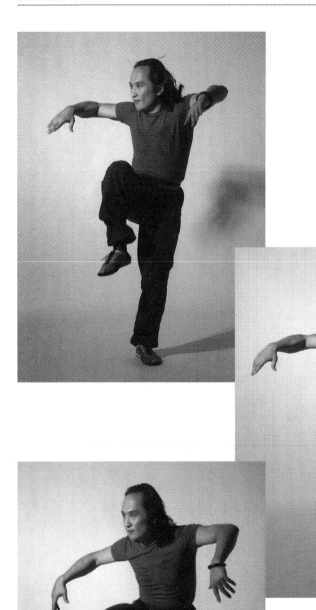

The joint must be like a spring in order to take the impact of landing

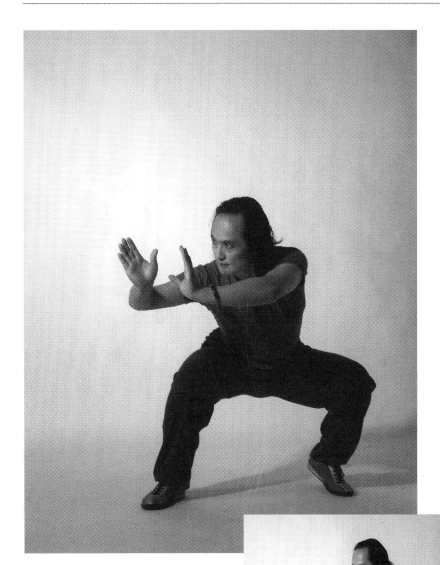

This is the son form from
'White ape offers fruit'

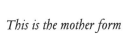

This is the mother form

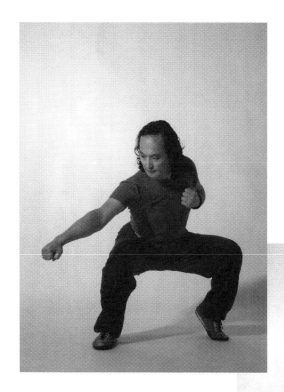

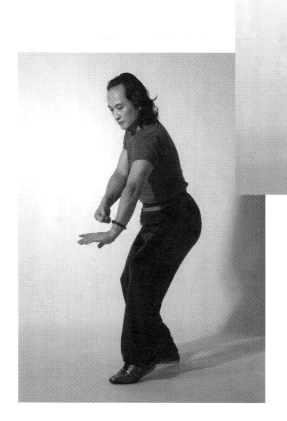

Hug the body, it needs to be very relaxed

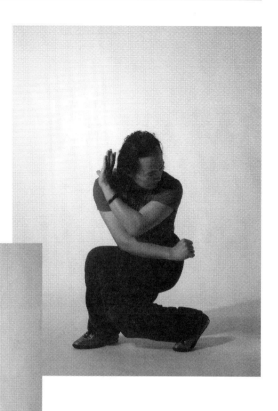

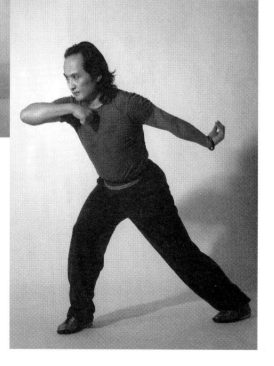

The closing and opening up of the body has a very distinct rhythm

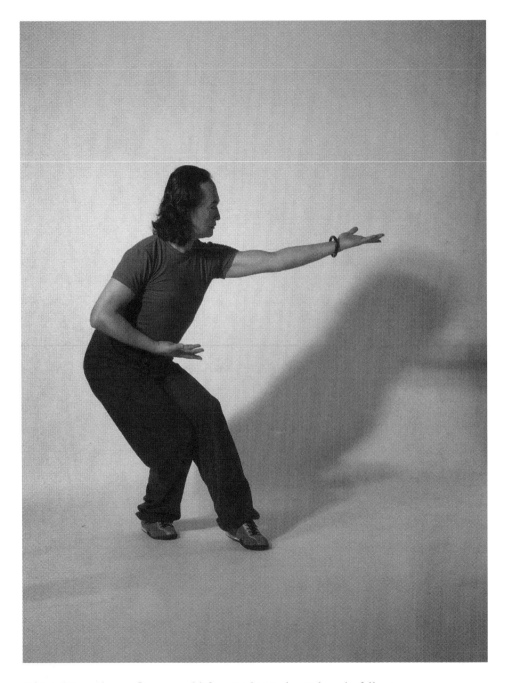

This is 'Green dragon flies upwards' from Eight Mother Palms; the following movements are derived from it

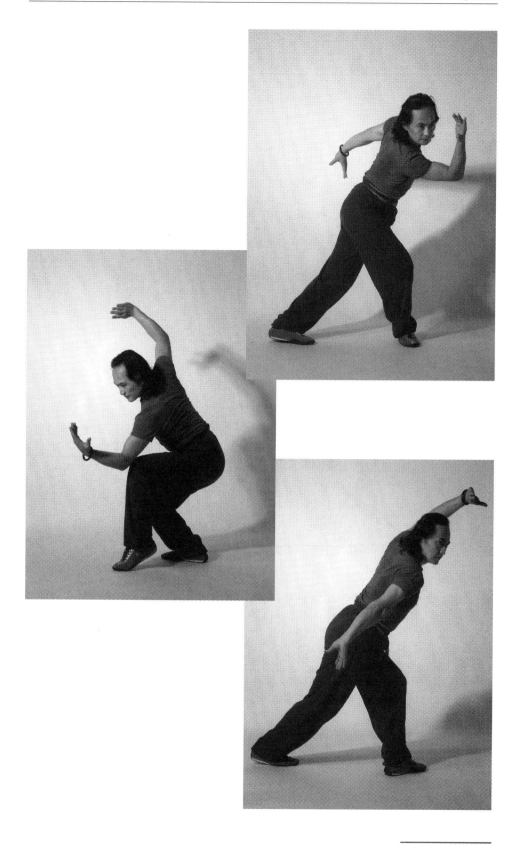

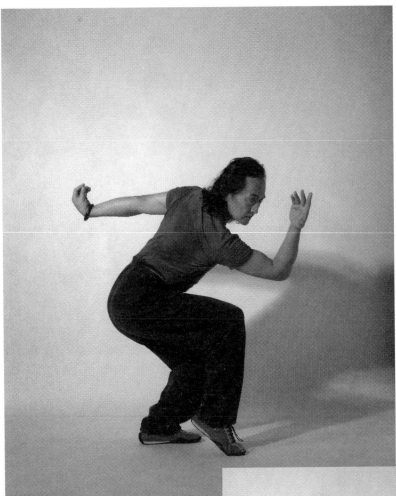

This is the son form from 'Green dragon flies upwards'

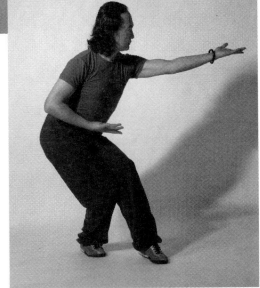

This is the mother form

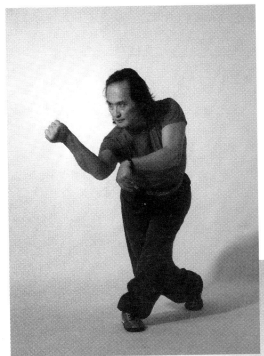

Looking for balance from unbalance produces a kinetic energy

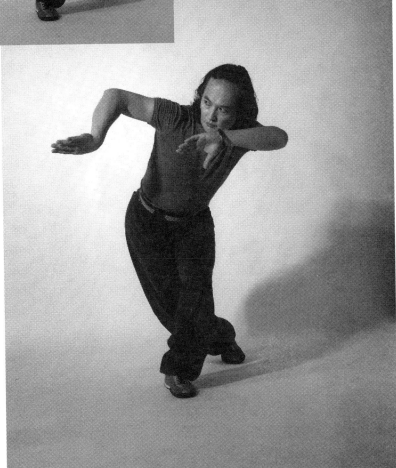

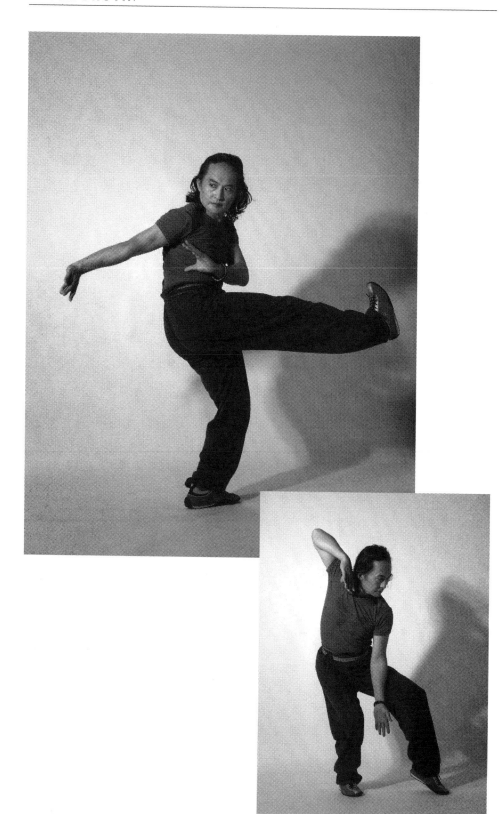

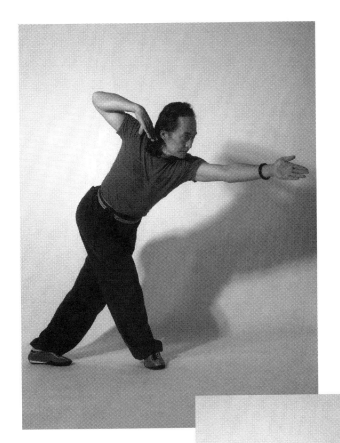

Does the body in this movement have some intersecting lines? Take a good look

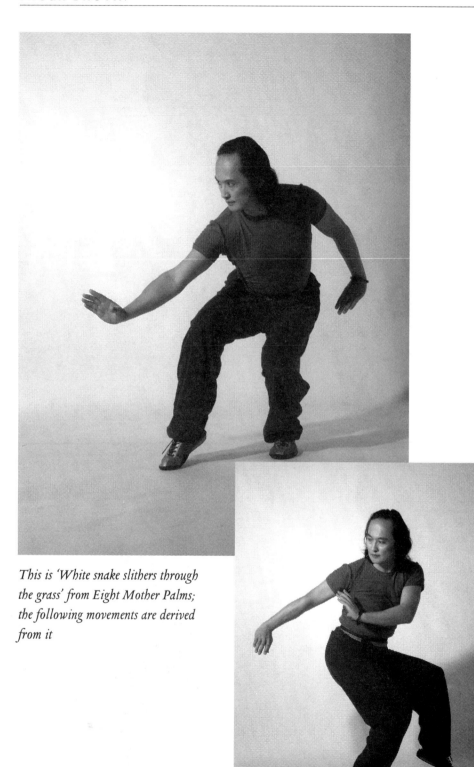

This is 'White snake slithers through the grass' from Eight Mother Palms; the following movements are derived from it

This is the son form from 'White snake slithers through the grass'

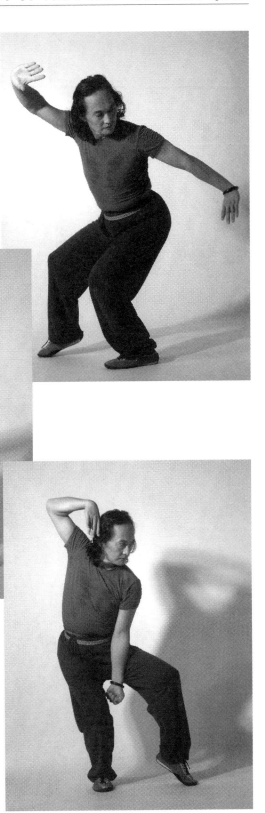

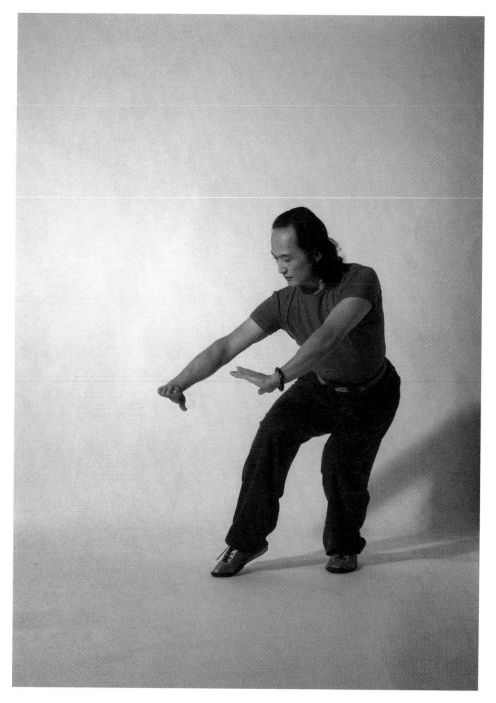

This is 'Chilin spits out the book' from Eight Mother Palms; the following movements are derived from it

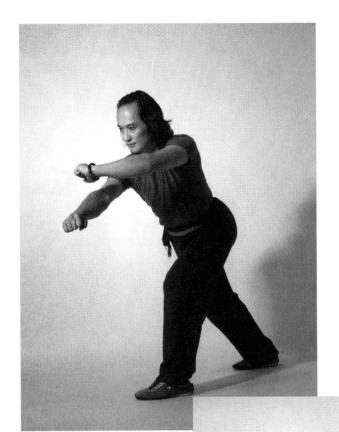

This is the son form from
'Chilin spits out the book'

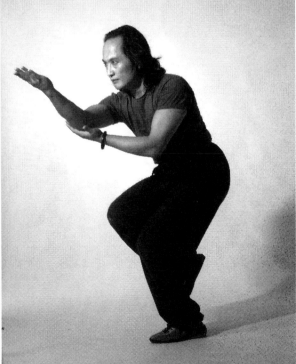

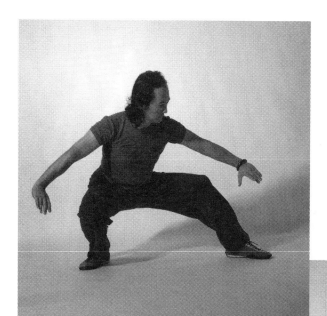

Closing posture

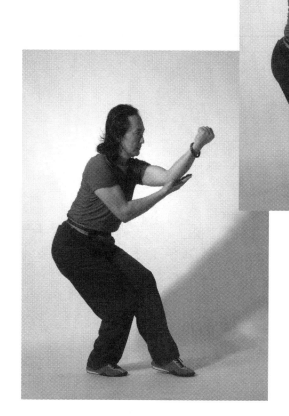

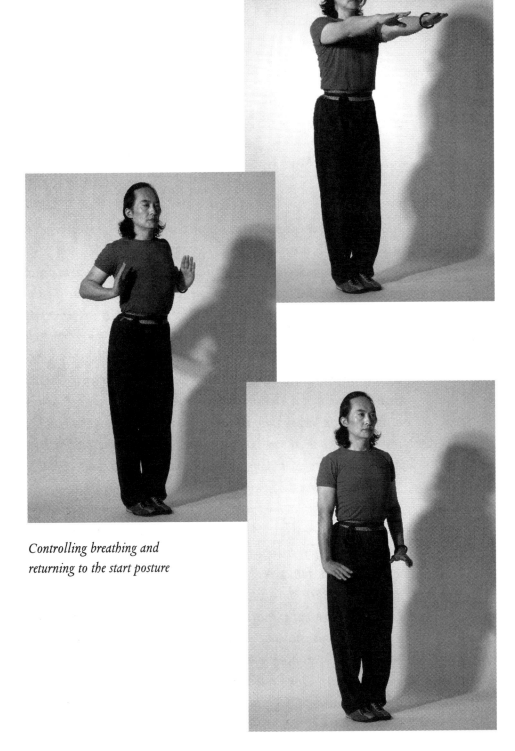

*Controlling breathing and
returning to the start posture*

CHAPTER 21

A Master's Confession

 A disciple once asked me: 'Master, you have lived for so long, what is man's life really all about?'

In an instant my life suddenly flashed before my eyes, not in detail or in sequence, but a faint taste came to root of my tongue. I said: 'Man's life, isn't it just to suffer?' In fact the family I was born into was not poverty stricken. It was a family of scholars; my elder uncle was a Qing government official and several other uncles were head-masters or schoolteachers. My father practiced traditional Chinese medicine and owned a medicine shop. In addition there were a number of silk spinning workshops in our home and of course we had quite a few fields. In short my family, which lived in Qingshan village, Mouping county, Shandong province, was a famous clan.

But then, since the family was too big and my parents too busy, I was from birth put in a separate room with a wet nurse. I only met my father a few times a year. When afterwards an disciple told me that I was not a good father I thought it over; I have studied many things in my lifetime but 'father' was a stranger to me from when I was small and had not been shown to me even by the time I was grown up. However I have had a 'master' which has also brought a master's wife, a grandfather master and a number of disciples. This has been my other family, even closer the original one.

My master, Gong Baotian, had been a fourth rank swordsman bodyguard at the Qing palace with the Yellow Riding Jacket, and practiced Bagua Quan. Afterwards he had retired and returned to his village where he lived by himself. The master's family was in Qingshan village and not prosperous, so he had little contact with others; villagers rarely met him and most people did not know him.

My physique was weak and sickly from the start; people who knew me all called me 'coffin fodder' since it did not look like I would live for long. I was lucky that my father was a traditional doctor and had his own medicine shop. I could take medicine every day and hung on to my life.

My elder uncle was a fourth grade Qing government official and was acquainted with the master. He saw that my physique was very weak and secretly passed me on to the master, hoping that Bagua Quan would improve my health and build up my strength. Since my family was scholarly and martial arts were looked down on, I did not want to say that I was practicing. Thinking about it I was about eight years old then.

It was probably from the age of eight or nine that I started studying during the day at home – the 'Three Trimetrical Classic', the 'One Hundred Family Names', the ancient classics (need I go on), the 'Fours Books and Five Canons' right down modern subjects such as mathematics, physics and chemistry; there was nothing I did not study. Since the house was full of scholars, there was no shortage of people to teach me. When evening came I would secretly go to a training room to practice Bagua Quan right up until past midnight and then secretly return to my room, change my sweat soaked clothes, take hold of a big lotus basin, clean myself with two ladlefuls of cold water and then go to bed. Several years passed, the four seasons as one. Nobody in the house knew I was training. These then were the days of my youth.

The village of Qingshan was surrounded by precipitous mountains. Day to day disputes with neighbouring villages over cultivation and water supply were unavoidable. It was a time of turmoil. Stragglers and disbanded soldiers were always gathering in the mountains. The village was surrounded all year round by hostile forces, ranging from triads and communist guerrilla bands to pro-Japanese traitors and communist troops. All generations of Qingshan's inhabitants struggled to survive – bravery was their natural trait.

The disciple said that I was not a good father. I asked: 'what is a good father?' The disciple replied: 'if there is a disagreement he should communicate and not rule autocratically'. To tell the truth that new expression 'communicate' does not yet exist in my brain. As I see it 'the elder is respected, the strong is the greatest'. The weak then must be obedient and so the one who obeys is the weak one. The bravery in Qingshan was a matter of strength not of ' communicating'. What on earth sense is there in a father obeying a son?

You see, from the age of eighteen or nineteen I started to be in charge of things. The clan was so big, there were so many businesses, so many adults and children, outside tenant farmers and partners, so much going on that if every matter had to be 'communicated', only half the work would have got done. So although I in fact understand this thing of 'communicating' it can't be done in an instant. On this point the disciple has confirmed that I really felt apologetic to my children and hoped that they could forgive me.

The generation gap between me and my children is also the gap between me and the present times. In my life I have experienced the most rapid change in the history of China. The historic changes of dynasty and government have not changed what is right and wrong, good and evil. But in my lifetime, thirty to forty years of upright living, and especially so in that twenty year period, right and wrong, good and evil, poverty and wealth, honour and disgrace, gain and loss, could overnight be reversed as one band of people came and another departed, one flag was hoisted and another lowered. There was nothing that could be hung on to, nothing that could be adhered to, nothing that could be believed in, nothing that could be hoped for. There was only yourself, only your own strength to meet the strain. And finally your speed in meeting the strain would be outpaced by the times.

I do not want you to think that I am a diehard, opposed to change. When I was in the prime of my life, aged forty-three to forty-four, I was the manager of two newspapers in Qingdao, 'Guanghua Daily' and 'Pingmin Daily', and also a reporter for the 'Zhongyuan News Agency'. At that time I wore western clothes and a western style top hat every day. This was the result of my single handedly making my living in the wide world for over ten years. There is no need for me to elaborate on the hardships – I had been hungry, poor, wounded and almost killed. But when the bitterness ends the sweetness begins. I had accumulated forty years of ability and ambition and finally a great expanse of sky had let me spread my wings and fly.

That afternoon in 1949, the thirty-eighth year of the Republic, I was walking along Qingdao Street. Something noisy was going on nearby, a disturbance in the market. Suddenly a man rushed across and grabbed me, shouting 'Baozhai, leave at once, the Eighth Route Army have entered the city. They won't let you stay free'. He thrust six silver dollars into my hand and dragged me through the crowds to the dock. I pushed my way on board a steamship and, before I knew it, I had left Qingdao, the city of my hopes. It was as if I had been knocked out before I had even seen the enemy, it was all over in a flash – happiness, anger, grief, enjoyment – all my feelings – left behind.

The communists would never have let me stay free. During the Japanese occupation I had shielded a guerrilla unit in Qingdao under the cover name 'Gong Yujun'. My wife was called 'Gong Linyu'. I didn't get on well with pro-Japanese traitors and communist forces. Afterwards I got a job as bodyguard to the teachers at the Laiyang No 6 United Middle School and could not help but have to fight communists inside and outside the school. This gradually intensified and gave me no option but to leave as soon as possible. (After the No 8 United Middle School was set up in Laiyang, the teachers and pupils of the No 6 United School moved their school to my home village of Qingshan. They carried tables and chairs along winding, tortuous roads, like a band of soldier ants.)

Although the changes that affect a man's life are beyond his control they are often his own choice. After Zhang Xiaogu of the Renmin Newspaper arrived in Taiwan he came to see me and said: 'Baozhai, I have brought a car with me. I will sell it, We will make a comeback and run a newspaper again.' However at that time I was down at heart. I had given up the scholarly way and the martial way. I was thinking of joining the guerrillas in the mountains. Afterwards I heard that the communists had burnt down the mountain vegetation cover and that the guerrillas had been forced out. All that could be done was send someone to pick up my wife and kids and return them to Taiwan where they could wait until the situation improved before returning to their homes. Who could know that I would still be waiting fifty years later, still having a son and daughter left at home.

I refused Zhang Xiaogu's invitation. Through my own efforts I became a locksmith. Using my skills in Bagua Quan I helped many refugees who had lost their keys to open locks. I earned a little money and opened the Gongji bicycle repair shop opposite Taipei's Nanmen market. Soon afterwards my son and daughter were born. The family still suffered from poverty and ill health and I was unable to make ends meet. After my wife gave birth she fell ill from a haemorrhage to the uterus – a basin of blood was lost. In the middle of the night I hired a three-wheeler taxi to rush her to hospital. The uterus had collapsed and she barely survived. In convalescence she had the right to eat eggs, but under children's hungry eyes, she always shared one egg with them.

I also caught TB and had the right to eat meat. The Taiwan sanatorium sent me home and told me to prepare to die. I was not going to admit defeat. Since retreating to Taiwan I had been powerless. Surely I should not throw away my own life. So I again took up Bagua Quan which I had practiced from childhood and after a string of defeats in my life I won a small victory.

As you can well imagine in the time that I had been in Taiwan my mood had been affected by the famous Shandong temper and I was not getting on well with my relatives. Afterwards I opened the Wanbao hardware shop in Wenchang street. Life gradually became better, the children gradually grew up and I gradually became older; the children one by one left home. I occasionally had some new students and Bagua Quan disciples came and went. In the end there was only my wife and myself keeping each other company.

You say that the reason for life isn't suffering? When you are young you struggle with all your might and suffering is inevitable. You are defeated and try again. You fall down and pick yourself up. Life is a struggle to survive. It is not easy to stand steady on your feet; you feel like resting and relaxing and you discover that life has no interest.

Life for the young has become easier and easier. I have become more and more estranged from life. Old friends are dying before me. New friends speak improper language. Children go out early and come back late. You don't get to meet people. You can't understand some of the things children say. You don't know what the plays on TV are all about. The remote control is difficult to work. What is life about? Why do we live?

China has experienced the most rapid changes in her history. I am exhausted and don't want to move. The park of the Sun Yat Sen Memorial Hall has not one tree on which you can hang yourself. Sticking out your tongue to frighten people is not right.

My wife must not die before me; I must go first; I must not be last.

Where has your master's wife gone?

Has your mother left hospital?

Who is that stranger? (the nurse hired to look after him)

Where is this?

Can it be my home?

Where has your mother gone?

She is coming, she is coming over.

What is your mother doing standing so far away? Tell her to come over

Where has my family gone, my father and mother?

Master Gong Baozhai was born on 2nd December in the Sixth year before the Republic (1905) and died on 25th April in the eighty-ninth year of the Republic (2000). This article has been composed from the fragments of his life that I found out during my twenty-two years with him. The life of a ninety-six-year-old man is of course more than this. Perhaps I asked too few questions for the master often said: 'These things are not worthy of mention'.

Written by He Jinghan, 2 May 2000

CHAPTER 22

A Brief Account of the Life of Master Gong Baozhai

Mr Gong Baozhai was a native of Qingshan village, Mouping county, Shandong province. He was born on 2nd February, six years before the republic (1905) and died on 25th April in the eighty-ninth year of the republic (2000) at the age of ninety-six.

Gong Baozhai was apprenticed to a Bagua Quan master at the age of eight (this was Gong Baotian who was a fourth rank chief bodyguard at the Qing court).

For about thirty years in a row he practiced martial arts from morning to dusk. In the war against Japan he had a post at the Shandong No 6 United Middle School. After the victory over Japan he managed the Damin and Pingmin newspapers in Qingdao in conjunction with legislative member Zhang Xiaogu. He can be said to have been the complete person, with both the scholarly and the martial ways, well versed in martial arts and matters of culture.

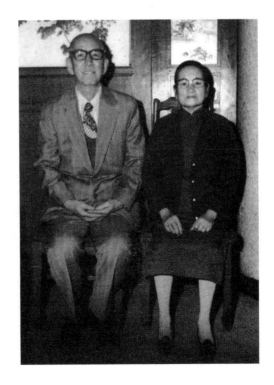

After coming to Taiwan, Master Gong lived a quiet life. He did not yield to Zhang Xiaogu's entreaties for him to return to newspaper management, but preferred to reconstruct his life through his own efforts. He became a locksmith, repaired bicycles and managed a hardware shop.

Master Gong was married for sixty-five years. Sadly his wife passed away on 25th January in the eighty-ninth year of the republic (2000). Master Gong, suffering from depression and exhaustion, followed her. The two were only apart for three months. It is a remarkable story.

Master Gong had the special responsibility of transmitting the treasures of Bagua Quan. His way of transmitting Bagua Quan was different from ordinary martial artists. He put the philosophy of martial arts first and combat second. He told his disciples to study calligraphy, ancient literature, chess and the philosophy of life, to seek to comprehend by analogy, to change their temperaments, to nurture restraint and modesty from within and to nurture a capacity in body and mind that had inner restraint and modesty and combined the scholarly and the martial ways. Master Gong's bequest of his treasure to his successors in Taiwan and America can be said to be his great contribution to human civilisation.

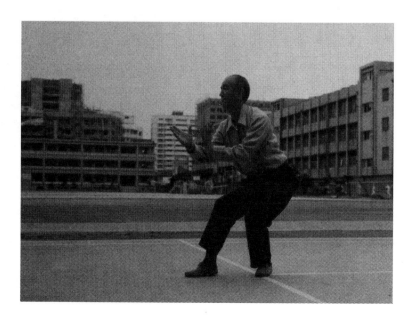

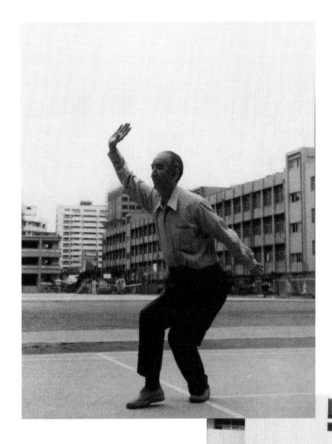

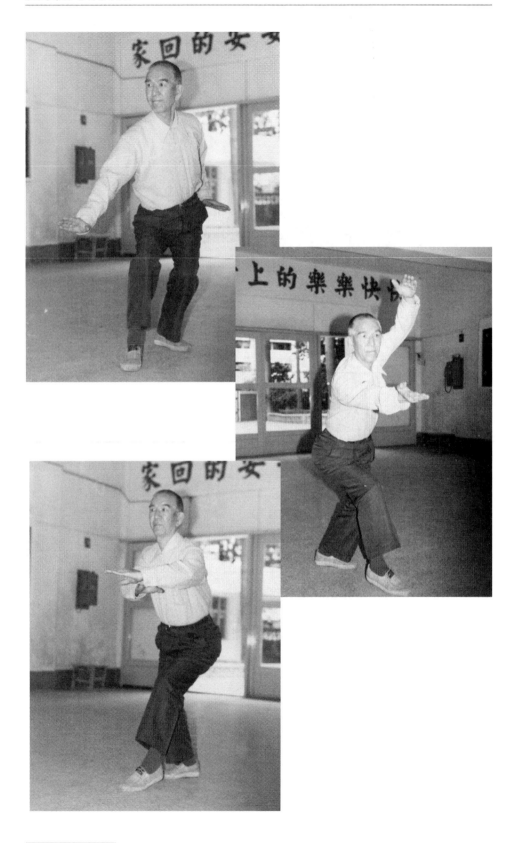

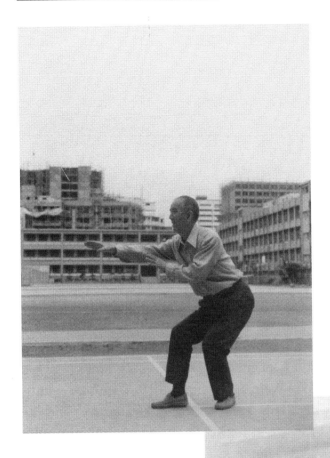

ABOUT THE AUTHOR

I was born on 9 January 1955 in a warehouse at No 1 wharf (Xinbin wharf) in the port of Gaoxiong. This was then a storehouse for military and government organisations and the families were separated by wooden partitions.

My father, He Weiran, was born in 1920 in Boai county, Hunan province. This was a poor and isolated area and life was hard. At the age of fourteen, when he was hardly taller than a rifle, he left home to join the army. Later on he attended the military district middle school and, in a hectic life, qualified for higher middle school where he graduated. In 1949 he came to Taiwan with the army and eventually

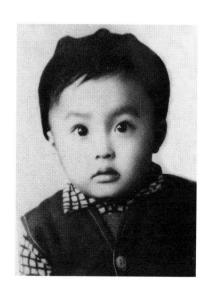

retired as a lieutenant colonel. He still studies calligraphy, painting and Taiji Quan – he does not admit defeat in his life or give in to old age.

My mother, Li Longyun, was born in 1931 in Kaifeng city, Hunan province. In 1948, a year before the mainland fell into enemy hands, in obedience to her parents' command she married a poor military man, my father, in order that she could be evacuated from the mainland with the army. Afterwards she raised four children in difficult times.

This was like growing four sturdy trees in a stony field by cultivating the soil over 30–40 years – it is hard to imagine. Although conditions at home were tough, growing up under the wings of my parents I never felt any hardship. Perhaps it is like the saying 'people born under Capricorn begin to understand things late, they are muddle headed and know nothing, but manage to do everything'. The most valuable things I have achieved in life have been like this – do not compete, do not fight, do not resist, it will happen by itself.

Probably it was father who encouraged us children to learn by heart the classics and the Three Hundred Tang dynasty poems. From when I was little I liked to write. After graduating from middle high school, although I chose to enlist in the army, my ambition at that time was still to become a writer.

A teacher at the middle high school, Yu Renlan, had a great influence on me. Although she perhaps did not know that she would influence me, the way of life that she instilled naturally guided the rebel that I was at that time.

Teacher Yu was born in 1915 in the northeast city of Jilin and graduated from the Sichuan Oriental Culture and Education Academy. From the age of seventeen she studied philosophy, Chinese national culture and calligraphy under the scholar Xia Puxu and at the age of eighteen she became a Buddhist. She never married. As a single, weak woman she took on the borderlands of education and offered her educational work as a tribute.

I was in teacher Yu's class in Qiangshu middle high school for three years. After graduation I still often asked her for advice right up to her death in 1987. My memory of teacher Yu is of her with her hair like noodles in a clear soup, dressed in a comfortable cheongsam in the modern style and a pair of flat black sneakers, a book always in her hand, writing on the blackboard one stroke at a time in regular script, talking not too fast and not too slow but with profound force. 'My aim of saving the nation and the people has not yet been achieved. I do not want to stay in heaven, I must return to this world to fulfil my uncompleted aim.' This was her testament. Teacher Yu Renlan was a very clear headed person, not especially dazzling, but very steadfast, very clear headed.

My master, Gong Baozhai, was a different sort of person; upright and worldly wise, strict but sharp witted. His was a life of struggle for survival in the jungle. He did not have the opportunity to fulfil his aspiration of saving the nation and the people. He could only in those turbulent times use his own ability to fight his way up from the lower levels of society and to survive. But he taught me to read 'The King of Teng's Council Chamber', to study that boldness of vision; to read the 'Louhou Chronicle', to study the deportment of warriors; to read 'The War Proclamation for Xu Jingye's Expedition against Wu Zhao', to study that harsh and severe work. He taught me to study Ling Xiangru, Zhu Geliang and Zhao Yun. The flame in his heart to save the nation and the people has not yet expired in mine.

I was twenty years in the army during which time I attended the Foreign Language School, the electronic warfare course, the Communication University's electronics faculty and other schools. On my own initiative in official and private time I translated the *National Military Dictionary of Electronic Warfare Terminology*. I attended a military Chinese cultural writers course and studied martial arts with a master. I was secretary to the Republic of China Martial Arts Association. I finally retired from the army with the rank of lieutenant colonel. Reading and studying became my habits. 'Forming the qualities of moral integrity' became part of my blood. After leaving the army I took the post of creative ideas coordinator at the Chuanshen Audiovisual Company. I produced many training videos and published books. At present I am general manager of the Digital Martial Arts Company. The flame that was in the master's heart is still burning in mine.

So I have been formed by the above four people who in succession have been at my side to nurture me. Is it possible for me to establish a clear moral character in my lifetime? Looking at the long line of people before me, will there in future be someone who will be able say that he was influenced by He Jinghan? This is beyond my control and does not concern me. However to be able to establish a clear moral character in one's lifetime is very satisfying – after all, you should not spend your life in idleness, isn't that true?

BY OPENING THE ART'S PORTAL
YOU ENTER THE MYSTERIOUS GATE OF THE BODY

I have been acquainted with Master He for three years. Over 1000 days – not a long time but also not a short time. However, getting to know Bagua Daoyin has been the start of my new life. In these new surroundings I am like a three-year-old – muddled and lacking discipline.

In fact I am a middle aged woman – forty pushing fifty and already in the change of life. I have always paid attention to my appearance and my health. I have always been eager to try out any keep fit or beauty treatment product and course on the market. My friends jokingly call me 'the white rat' since I will nibble anything; they tell me about something new and encourage me to be the first to try it. But I could never stick with things and after half an hour's frenetic effort I would have a change of mind.

Faced with a body suffering from the ravages of time I often woke up at night in tears. My checkups with the doctor were all OK, it was just that looking after my health was not keeping pace with getting old. Where could I find the means of explaining the profound mysteries of my body which did not depend on external methods of health care? But, as the proverb says 'Providence does not let you down if you do your best'. I finally came across Bagua Daoyin.

It overturned my previous lifestyle and attitude to life. The teacher's training was in direct contrast to the usual methods of dividing up the class into beginner, intermediate and high levels, or selling you the myth that you can reach an effective standard in no time at all. The teacher made it clear to me that there was no way that my physical condition could be improved with just a few days of set exercise forms. Only by making my body the most important undertaking in my whole life and putting in a continuous effort could I change my physiological, psychological and even intellectual perceptions and thereby achieve real improvement. There was no trickery or shortcuts, only relying on myself to do repeated exercises, again and again. It was learning through practice with lots of sweat and not being afraid of pain. The days and months passed by quickly and produced results.

Bagua Daoyin especially emphasizes the perception and training of muscles, bones and skin. Every external movement is correlated to and echoed in the inner tissue of the body. Many bodies are uncomfortable due to poor posture. Take the very common occurrence of backache – we usually take medicine, have a massage or even use mechanical appliances to try to cure it. However, it is a mistake to feel that the only benefit in this situation comes from external forces; standing, sitting and lying postures are with us all the time. Some people spend two hours a week correcting the vertebrae but in the other twenty-two hours and six days treat their body in the old way. What good is that?

Within a short time of starting Bagua Daoyin, I found that my old body had become like a stranger to me, so much so that I could not use important joints. In this period the teacher taught me how to:

- put my head on my shoulder

- walk without using my legs

- relax when standing upright

- hunch my back without bending the waist

- kick like an ox even when I was not angry, and walk up and down stairs gracefully

Good Heavens! Did I really have to learn how to do all these things? But it was really difficult to learn how to do them because of all habits which I had unconsciously acquired and had to change. How easy is that?

In order to really change my movements I had to put in a big effort, going from practicing twenty minutes a day to practicing two hours a day come rain or shine. I threw away my rose coloured glasses and my routine of only putting in half an hour of frenetic practice. To my surprise I became a hardworking, persevering, conscientious 'bad' student. I was always making demands of the teacher. 'Teacher, do it again, I don't understand', although the teacher had already demonstrated it over ten times. 'Teacher, I don't understand your explanation, can you put it another way?'; 'I still can't understand, is there another way of doing it?'. After three years of really strenuous study like this my appearance has changed, my stamina is better than it was when I was thirty. I have gained about five centimeters in height, my waist and buttocks are trim and my muscles have filled out and are rounded and elastic. I can quickly recover from backache or colds. Most people don't believe my true age. I can still see my expression without looking in the mirror; I have radically changed my former ways of looking at people and things. It is easy to concentrate my mind. Practices that I previously could not do or did not understand have now suddenly come together, even though I have not yet got beyond the rudimentary level.

I can't help asking how come such a marvelous 'quintessence of Chinese culture' is known about by so few people. Isn't it true that 'virtue does not stand alone; it must be shared by many'? I have thought about it deeply for a long time. Originally it was because the teacher and other teachers continued to follow the tradition that the old saint keeps his virtue, remains hidden in mountains and forests, does not seek to spread the word, does not seek fame and wealth; that those who wish to learn will ask; that the martial arts master will only offer to teach if asked to do so.

It is very disappointing to see that Bagua Daoyin, this marvelous product of man, is disappearing. What a tremendous loss this would be for us all. So no matter what, this unique branch of martial arts knowledge must continue to flourish. We should take advice from all sides on how it can be developed in line with present day needs and teaching methods so that even more people can enjoy this great feast of the body and mind.

– Yan Lin
Executive Head of Bagua Daoyin Development Association

25 NOVEMBER 1999

At dusk on 25th November 1999 I was taking my usual stroll in the park of the Sun Yat Sen Memorial Hall when I suddenly saw in the corner of an avenue a gentleman practising Taiji Quan by himself. I glanced at him. The Taiji Quan he was practising was completely different from anything I had previously seen. It was full of strength and beauty yet had a continuous, unbroken power. I couldn't bear just to stand and watch. I waited until he had finished then went over to say hello. He replied very amiably and after a brief exchange of greetings I expressed an interest in learning. He quickly agreed and with this began my second life with Taiji Quan.

I had studied Taiji Quan more than twenty years previously, but only on and off due to pressure of work, and then other things had taken over. When I again had some leisure time I had thought of taking it up but it had been impossible to find a good teacher. Finally, after years of searching, my wish was being granted.

After starting lessons I realised that although the teacher's Taiji Quan was excellent, his Bagua Quan was something exceptional. What is more he was a fifth generation master of it. In every lesson he taught me some basic Bagua Quan movements to open up the joints of the body and relax the muscles. I realised that he had linked up the two branches of martial arts and had deeply probed into the body's secrets. It was a pleasure having a lesson with this teacher. I was able every time to feel the body's inner energy. Not only that but without being aware of it the teacher often showed a special but seldom met attitude to life which I admired very much.

Time rolled by and in a flash two years have passed. Although I still think of myself as a beginner the teacher has enabled me to become acquainted with my body.

Teacher He's book will enable his knowledge and teaching to benefit more and more people. I feel moved by his goodness of heart and his enthusiasm and devotion to martial arts. I hope that more and more friends will have the same good fortune as I and become acquainted with this great teacher of the body – Mr He Jinghan.

– Wang Shuyi
Chairman of Beian Rotary Club
Director of Qiren Middle School

A REMARKABLE MAN, A GOOD BOOK

I like reading. Not just works of literature but anything under the sun is my reading material. The Indian philosopher Rabindranath Tagore said 'What is known to mankind is like the dawn mist but the secrets of the universe are like the black night, immeasurably deep'. Then let me aspire to take the universe as my classroom and all things of creation as my teacher. I use reading to train my mind, I use reading to nurture my mind.

Since I like reading I chose to become a publisher. Although the work of a publisher is mentally stimulating it is not so active as other professions. So as I grew older, although I just about managed to keep my mind well organised, my body was going downhill and I was not able to do as much as I would have liked.

I felt that my colleagues were in the same position – advancing years exhausting the spirit. Through a friend I was introduced to teacher He Jinghan. In the first session he taught us all a number of exercises to move the joints. In that short lesson everyone realised that teacher He was an exceptional person. I then took a series of lessons with him. I started from a position of knowing nothing about Chinese martial arts and also was not very confident – I had not thought of myself as suitable material for martial arts training. I gradually had to reduce training due to work commitments and eventually gave up lessons with teacher He.

This was several years ago. When teacher He finished this book on his teaching and was preparing it for publication I had the good fortune to be able to read the manuscript. I opened the title page 'To open the micro-universe of the human body, to establish a universal concept of human life'. These words immediately led me to read on and discover the profound truth that seeking a way to peace of spirit while ignoring the basic philosophy of body and mind is like 'Attending to trifles while neglecting the essentials'. I read 'Freedom and ease start with the body'; 'If a person cannot master his body and mind it will be difficult for him to become an integrated person'. The teacher wrote 'Using fine movements to train the body and mind is the first step to learning the unity of the body and mind' and 'For true tranquillity of mind you must first regulate your body and then train for calmness amidst chaos, calmness amidst temptation, calmness amidst stimulation. Only then will you be able to achieve true, solid and beneficial tranquillity of mind'; 'If you can attain the state of harmony and balance over the long term, not only will you have a healthy body and mind you will also have a happy life'. Was this not the state for which I had been yearning and striving?

This is a really good book. Every concept in it can change your life. It is like the legendary bag of martial arts secrets with the difference that you do not need to 'fly over the eaves, walk on walls and steal treasures from the pavilion at night'. You can buy it in an ordinary bookshop. Teacher He is truly remarkable person.

A remarkable man, a good book. I have had the pleasure of reading it and I have greatly benefited from the experience. I extend my sincere respects to the author.

– Jian Zhizhong
Chairman of Yuangshe Publishing House

THE KEY TO OPENING UP THE BODY – BAGUA DAOYIN

The twenty-first century is an age of spiritual awakening. As life enters this brand new dimension, consciousness requires an ever higher level of sensitivity and clarity. The body is the mirror of the soul. It reflects an individual's inner spiritual state, the extent of our spiritual harmony, the extent to which we have activated our health.

With the many-sided, hectic lives most people live today, the basic unity of the body has been broken by pressure on the spirit, loss of the qualities of time and peace of mind, and the immersion of the body, mind and spirit in the battlefield of confusion and conflict. The body has begun to lose its original balance, to prematurely age, to grow senile. What is heartening is that when consciousness begins to acquire awareness, a way out appears. The body is a very direct and fast way to transform consciousness. Bagua Daoyin is an extremely effective way of opening up the body's intelligence. Its simple methods can thoroughly and reliably change long engrained habits of the body and restore the body's elasticity and harmony.

The first time I met teacher He Jinghan I was seven months pregnant with my second son. In teacher He's profound expression I saw the bearing of a martial art's inheritor, upright and determined but with the unconventional flavour of a layman. At that moment the baby in my womb gave a kick and I felt that the baby was telling me that my body needed some changes. We decided on the spot to study Bagua Daoyin with teacher He, and two months after the birth I started a Bagua Daoyin course with my elder son Hanning.

In training under teacher He's expert guidance we were able to deeply experience the systematic awakening of the body's lost sensitivity and awareness. With simple body movements we channelled the hidden flow of Qi, giving a new lease of life to the zones of the body that had lost their vitality – it was just like new shoots blooming on a withered tree. Teacher He assigned us body movements according to our individual physical condition and adapted his instruction to the individual student's level. You have only to maintain awareness and practice these exercises continuously in your daily life, to unlock the keys to the body's intelligence and thereby awaken the body and give it greater freedom. The mood of the body will become calmer and happier and the mind freer and more at ease. Only when you are whole-heartedly focused can you temper yourself and bring the world under your control. Great aspirations to change the world must come from purifying your own body and soul. A thousand foot tall tree is not far from its roots. A hundred flowers that bloom are not far from the heart – all things in creation return to their roots.

We believe that exploring this book will open up a new dimension in your life.

– You Mingyu and Wang Tingyu
Founders of the Xinlinghai Educational Establishment